The Joy of Eating

*The Anti-Diet Solution for
Weight Loss and Health*

Gwen Irwin

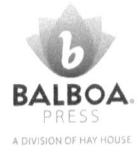

BALBOA
PRESS

A DIVISION OF HAY HOUSE

Balboa Press books may be ordered through booksellers or by contacting:

Balboa Press
A Division of Hay House
1663 Liberty Drive
Bloomington, IN 47403
www.balboapress.com
1 (877) 407-4847

Print information available on the last page.

ISBN: 978-1-5043-6051-7 (sc)
ISBN: 978-1-5043-6052-4 (e)

Balboa Press rev. date: 09/14/2016

To my niece Sarah who inspires me to be a better person and to keep writing.

Acknowledgements

Thank you to my friends and family for supporting this dream, thanks to Ken and Rebecca for huge editing help, thanks to Deb for proofreading and keeping me sane throughout this process, thanks to Phil for walking me through some freak-out moments, thanks to Andy for believing in me and helping me hold a high vibration, and thanks to the folks at Balboa press for making this dream a reality.

Table of Contents

Chapter 1

My Mom Died and I'm Worried about Being Fat

My mom died suddenly and unexpectedly from a massive stroke 12 years ago. I was devastated. And I was furious with myself and devastated a second time because I was fat.

One of my best friends from childhood came right away to help me with the arrangements. I told her we had to go shopping because I had nothing to wear to the wake and funeral. We went to the crappy mall and I hunted through the plus sized racks for a couple of black outfits that didn't make me look like hell.

I said to Sue, "Of course I have to be fat right now when I'm going to see all these people I haven't seen in years." Nice perspective. I was devastated, sad—and fat.

But I felt that way. On top of being a wreck because I would never see my mother again, sad beyond measure about losing her, terrified about the thought of my ailing father living alone three hours away, I also felt mortified to see old friends.

I was bigger than I had ever been. When I lived in my home town of Pittsfield, MA I was pretty consistently thin. I certainly was well into my dieting roller coaster ride by the time I left, but at that time I was more often in a thin cycle than a fat one, and I hadn't yet dieted myself up to my current weight.

How awful—at this time, when I needed to be grieving my mother and soaking in the warmth and love of old friends who came to support me, I was instead consumed with what they would think of me, as well as with my complete self-loathing. I was sure they would silently judge me for having gained so much weight, and I thought maybe I would have had a boyfriend or husband to stand with me in the surreal receiving line if I wasn't fat.

I begin with this story because I want you to know what held me back for years from losing my excess weight—our beliefs, thoughts, and words create the reality we see before us, a phenomenon that has come to be known as the law of attraction. Whether we are aware of it or not it is a law, just like the law of gravity, and it is working in our lives all the time. Did you notice the way I was talking and thinking about myself? That negative self-talk wasn't just because of this extraordinary circumstance of my mom's death—that was the way I talked about myself all the time.

I have not come across anyone who longs to be overweight! And when we are, a good majority of us believe beating ourselves up about it is a requirement. We think, *I will shame myself into losing weight. I will let everyone else know that I know I'm fat—I know I have to get myself back on a diet. I will say it aloud to others because I know they are thinking it.*

What a dreadful place to live. Then, when I consider the truth of *thoughts create reality,* I can see why none of my weight loss efforts were ever successful. Nearly all I thought and talked about was how fat I was and what diet I was on or about to go on.

Ever since I started struggling with weight and diet right out of elementary school, I've had a deep longing to find a sustainable solution; a longing to help others who are in a constant battle against their bodies, because I know how consistently heartbreaking it is.

I am truly grateful to have finally found a solution. And it began with stopping dieting and changing my excessively negative thoughts and dialog about food, diet, and my body.

This is the critical piece that is missing when it comes to sustainably losing weight—if you don't change the way you think about food and yourself, your efforts at weight loss will inevitably be thwarted.

You will continue to attract solutions that don't work for you, or if you find a solution that seems to be working and makes you feel better, you will talk yourself out of continuing with it.

So if you are struggling and miserable about the way you look and feel, before looking for yet another diet solution stop and really pay attention to your thoughts and words around food, diet, and your body. What are your beliefs around why you gained the weight—do you berate yourself for your lack of willpower, feeling like a bad person for "letting" this happen? What are your beliefs about having to be on a diet—do you believe you have no control over yourself around food? Where is that out-of-control feeling coming from? When you start to look at these negative thoughts and beliefs, you may see that it's not you who is out of control, but how strict the diet is that's causing these feelings.

Our thoughts create an endless cycle of angst and weight gain. It's time to stop—stop torturing and start nourishing ourselves.

******

There are a lot of things that cause us stress here on planet Earth. But the one thing I see that causes more suffering for more people than almost anything else is their relationship with food and weight.

The diet industry is one of the biggest industries in the world, supported by millions of people unhappy with their bodies and fearful about what to eat. You can't stand in line at the grocery store without seeing at least one new diet in the magazines that line the checkout. I say "at least" because usually there are several. What are the implications of this?

One implication is that there is something wrong with most of us—that we are not the right shape or size. And what should we do about it? Go on this new miracle diet—it really works!

My story about food and weight is a long one, as is the case for so many people. My foray into the world of dieting and fear of food started just out of elementary school. I had always been a skinny kid, tall and lanky, and I ate whatever I wanted—and I ate a lot! But as I entered junior high I felt awkward, ugly, and like I just didn't fit in. I figured there must be something wrong with me.

I concluded that what was wrong with me was my body and that I needed to lose some weight. It's so sad because that was the last thing I needed to do. But I decided that all of these magazines and ads on TV couldn't be wrong so I found a book called *Thin Thighs in Thirty Days*.

That book was so full of hope and promise for me. I had found the problem—my big thighs. I thought, *How can I possibly fit in with these giant thighs? Who is going to like me when I look like this? My life is really going to take off once I get this thigh situation under control. This is the answer!*

I diligently followed the program, speed walking around my neighborhood like a nut. I sweated through the various

5

forms of leg lifts and obediently followed the low calorie diet, eating as little as I could without alarming my parents. I was starving all the time but I lost weight—yay!

OK, not really yay. The reality was that I became too thin, looking almost ill. Eventually, I got to the point where I couldn't stand the restrictive diet any longer, and went back to eating like a normal twelve-year-old. But it was too late—what I had actually done was set myself up for about three decades of dieting and losing weight, only to gain it back plus some each time. When I got into my forties I had dieted myself into obesity—size 22 on a good day. But what is sadder than that is I had constant anxiety and fear about eating food.

As humans we are endowed with a sense of taste. We also need food to survive. So I am guessing that eating was supposed to be a pleasing sensory experience. Boy have we mucked that up! For so many of us, eating turns into a fear-based and unpleasant experience. We are either "being good" by denying ourselves sustenance, and likely starving a lot of the time, or "being bad" by eating something we enjoy but think will cause us to gain weight. It is a constant battle that we never win and we end up fearing the very thing that sustains us!

Dieting and weight "issues" are so commonplace that they seem normal to us. Food and weight are constantly on so many of our minds. It takes up a lot of time and energy. I never realized how much time and energy until I quit dieting!

It took me a long time to get to that realization though. After my plunge into the dieting world with the Thin Thigh program I tried just about every diet out there. Each magazine with the latest fad offered new hope and the promise of a better life once I got a handle on this weight problem (that I, of course, had created all on my own!). Each time I started anew there was energy behind it, but I now know that energy was driven by fear. And the fear became greater and greater as I ultimately gained more and more weight.

Every day on a diet started with the scale, and the number on the scale would set my mood for the day. There was the fleeting euphoria when the numbers were going down, and then the sheer panic and self-hatred when they were going up. So much of my life revolved around that number.

There was the constant agonizing about food—what I would eat, whether I would let myself eat, and then all the self-judgment around whatever I decided to do. Of course, all this thinking led to me talking about it a lot, which was easy to do because so many people had the same feelings and fears around food, diet, and body image. Even friends who I considered quite thin talked about diets and weight. It didn't take any effort to get a conversation going, and I never realized how much I talked about it until I stopped talking about it.

Despite all the studying and reading I had done over the last 25 years about how we manifest things into our lives, I just wasn't getting it that my thoughts, words, and beliefs were the reason I stayed in this perpetual cycle of losing and gaining weight, and living with all the fear that surrounds it. I guess I thought weight was somehow exempt from the law of attraction.

******

The last time I lost weight (and then gained it back plus) on a diet was after my mom died. I was determined, after feeling the way I had after she passed, that I was going to take the weight off. I still had the mentality that something was wrong with me and that losing weight by following yet another diet would fix it. A friend at work suggested we go to Weight Watchers—we could go at lunch time.

As usual, I started out with great zeal. Instead of counting calories or fat grams, Weight Watchers assigns a point value to all foods. I was an excellent point counter! I always wanted to save a few points for wine so I was not eating much and what I was eating consisted mostly of frozen diet dinners—that way I could be sure about the points. What I was consuming was basically void of nutrients but that fact never even crossed my mind. Once again, I was able to force some of the weight off, and once again I was starving all the time, which left me perpetually on the edge of anger. I remember vowing *I will never do this again,* meaning gain back the weight and have to go on another diet and feel the way I felt. I started gaining the weight back before I even got to my goal.

The panic I felt as the weight began to creep back up was palpable. I had to buy bigger clothes. Each new size instilled terror in me to the point where I freaked out on the cute, young sales girl at the Banana Republic outlet. I searched every rack just to find that they only carried up to a size 14. I knew the regular Banana carried 16, which at that time was my current bodily manifestation. My friend persuaded me to ask and when she answered, "No, I'm sorry, we don't carry anything above a 14," I practically yelled, "That's discrimination!" She replied in a very kind way, "I know, that's what my mom says."

I cannot overstate how strong my feelings of panic were. I was living my life from this place of fear. As I said, what an awful place to live.

Even after my weight started to creep back up it still took me some time to see that what I was doing wasn't working on so many levels. I continued to gain weight and to hate myself for it. Finally, I got to a breaking point. I couldn't stand feeling this way any longer and having so much judgment towards myself. It was just cruel. If anyone else had said the things to me that I was saying to myself and about myself I would have been devastated. Something had to change.

The pain of living with all that fear and self-loathing finally became greater than the pain of being overweight. I made the decision to quit dieting—for GOOD. I had tried that a couple of times before but I got too frightened because my belief in having to be on a diet to lose weight was so strong. Finally, I could no longer deny the fact that dieting made me ultimately gain more weight.

I quit all diet foods. I didn't count anything—points, calories, or fat grams. I ate when I was hungry and stopped when

I was full. But more important than all of that, I stopped saying mean things to myself and about myself. I did not engage in any type of diet talk. And I began to make peace with food.

It was one of the best things I have ever done in my life! First of all, I realized how much time and energy I spent thinking and worrying about food and my weight. It was exhausting! And I realized that I rarely enjoyed eating, even when eating my favorite foods, because I had so much guilt around eating them. When I was on a diet I was happy when I got to eat and convinced myself that I liked the processed frozen foods I was eating, but I wasn't by any means nourishing myself. The feeling of being almost constantly hungry, sometimes feeling starved, really wore me down, physically and emotionally. I was barely getting my needs met on a most basic level.

Allowing myself to eat what I wanted when I was hungry was such an amazing and liberating thing. It sounds so weird to say, "Allowing myself to eat." I am incredibly fortunate to live in a part of the world where food is abundant and I am also very fortunate to have the means to buy good quality food. Yet, despite that, I had for years been making the choice to go hungry much of the time.

My guilt around eating didn't go away immediately, but as my weight stabilized I began to calm down. It was such a pleasure to be open to all the possible food choices, decide what I was in the mood for, and then eat it! It was so empowering to stop eating when I felt full, to no longer have anxiety that I couldn't eat a certain food again. I "trained" myself to stop eating when I was full by continually assuring myself that, even if one minute after I put what remained of my meal in the refrigerator I felt like I was still hungry or wanted more, I could pull it back out and continue eating. Even if I only had a couple of bites left of whatever I was eating I still wrapped it up and put it in the fridge.

My coworker used to laugh at what she found in the refrigerator, but it was a successful strategy nonetheless. Now I am at the point where if there are only a couple of bites left I can throw it out. Sometimes I will let it sit on the counter for a little while before throwing it out if I am not absolutely sure I am done. All of this may sound silly or weird, but it was so important during this learning process.

And that is what this was—the process of learning a new habit. The power of habit energy is amazing. My habit was dieting. It came about from my belief that I didn't fit in and that belief was strengthened with each weight loss and subsequent gain. Even though the cycle kept repeating itself and always ended poorly (in fact worse each time) I kept looking to the same "solution". I couldn't seem to look outside of the box because I believed in the box so much.

Once, while still deep in this habit energy, I went to a bookstore with a good friend who was pregnant and wanted to pick up a couple of books on what to expect. She was excited as this was her first child. Instead of sharing in her joy, I, in full weight gain mode, broke off from her and went straight to the diet section. I remember the visceral feeling of panic as I combed through the books for something new, something I hadn't seen before. The answer HAD to be there. I HAD to find it. I felt completely desperate. That day there was nothing new on the shelves, nothing I hadn't already tried. But that knowledge didn't shake me up enough to break the habit energy and shift the way I behaved. Unsuccessful at finding a new book, I just went back to one of the many diets I had already tried, thinking it would finally work. *I must not have tried hard enough last time.*

As painful as all those years of dieting were, there was also something comforting about it—dieting was familiar. The cycle was known and the process was wired into my brain. To quit dieting sounds so simple and like something everyone would want to do. No one I have ever talked to *likes* being on a diet. But the fear around not being on a diet, which fuels this familiar habit, is so great for so many people that they can't get back to seeing food as something that nourishes and sustains them.

So, quitting dieting was indeed a learning process and something I had to literally train myself to do. Science now shows that in order to break a habit and form a new one, you have to form new neuro pathways in your brain. It takes time and consistency to make a new way of being feel familiar and comfortable. It amazes me as I look back on my own shift that a lot of the things that feel comfortable to us cause us so much pain. I am grateful beyond words that I was finally able to push through all the fear I had about giving up this habit to get to the place I am in today.

******

There I was, bucking the diet system. Initially it was really uncomfortable. My weight stabilized but it stabilized at the highest it had ever been. That was the next piece—I had to accept it. I had to accept my body exactly the way it was and continue on with what I was doing. I had to accept what other people might think of me—an obese person eating non-diet, full-fat food. I had to learn to be OK with the fact that I was moving away from a belief in dieting that so many people clung to so tightly. I had to change my own belief amidst the collective belief.

This was an interesting process—accepting myself even though I wasn't generally accepted by society. There were occasional comments (not aimed directly toward me) about "fat people". Regardless, I stayed the course. I didn't cave and go back to my comfort zone—dieting and engaging in all things diet related. I stuck with it long enough to start blazing some new neuro pathways in my brain.

I cannot express how freeing it was to just eat. Just eat. Eat what I wanted when I wanted. Eat without guilt. Eat real food. Just *eat*. I cannot express how good it felt to have so much time and energy freed up. Thinking about food, worrying about food, feeling guilty about food, beating myself up about food—that takes a lot of time and energy. And it doesn't feel good!

This is how my journey of getting back to myself and my naturally thin size began and how it HAD to begin. If I hadn't changed my thoughts and beliefs about food, diet and body image, and accepted myself exactly the way I was, no matter what I did with regard to diet, exercise, or nutrition it never would have worked.

I spent many years in this space of acceptance and peace around food. I still had the desire to lose my excess weight, but instead of feeling desperate what seemed to me a miracle occurred. I developed a strong feeling deep inside me that the weight would somehow come off organically, without a struggle.

******

Through a series of seemingly random events, the organic solution I knew would show up fell right into my lap! *Seemingly random.* I found a healthy eating style that made me feel great, that was totally satisfying, and with no struggle at all the weight started to take care of itself.

What empowered me to be able to find my own healthy way of eating was to make peace with food and accept where I was minute to minute. If you struggle with fear around food, diet, and body image, and subsequently with your weight and health, my hope is to help you find the joy of eating, to make peace with food and find a way of eating that you love and that gets you back to health and your naturally thin self. And in the midst of this process I think you will find that peace will spill into other areas of your life. Eat good food; feel good about what you eat. That is my wish for you.

Chapter 2

Eat Good Food; Feel Good about What You Eat

I often check Google analytics to see what keywords people are searching to get to my website. I should be doing this to strategize on my search engine optimization plan, but really I do it because it often cracks me up. One day, I came upon a phrase that really struck me: *fat, sick, and feeling dead inside.*

I don't know if this person meant to input the movie title *Fat, Sick, and Nearly Dead* and messed it up, which would be funny in my book. But I wondered, *Is somebody out there really feeling dead inside because they are overweight and sick?* Not so funny.

Nobody, in my experience, wants to be fat—it sucks! It's tiring, it's uncomfortable, and being overweight can also bring a long list of health problems. So not only is the overweight upsetting, the aching joints and stomach problems, among other things, add to the dismay.

Recent statistics show that in the US 68.5% of adults are overweight or obese; 34.9% are obese.

Wow, those numbers are huge, but I'm not surprised.

I'm not surprised but I am kind of incensed. Not because so many people are overweight, but *why* they are overweight.

The reason is this: The diet industry has us duped. Artificial sweeteners, diet "foods", light, low fat, no fat. When we are overweight we are told to go on a diet—count calories, count points, count fat grams, count carbohydrates. Meal plans filled with artificial foods are designed to fit the bill.

All of this processed and artificial food is keeping the majority of the United States overweight. We are getting a lot of bad information about what to eat and we need to turn it around.

The key to weight loss and health is so simple it's like it is hidden in plain sight. Here it is: Eat real food. Don't starve yourself or go on a diet that is not sustainable. Eat lots of nutrient-dense vegetables. Eat whole foods.

When you get on the path of eating whole, nutrient-dense food your cravings for processed faux foods will start to dwindle. In the meantime your body will get the nutrients it needs and the weight and health issues will start to take care of themselves.

But there is another problem the diet industry creates that will trip us up even if we get on the whole food path. In addition to giving us a lot of bad information and processed diet "foods", it has us programmed to feel lousy about ourselves at any weight, and to feel extreme guilt when we eat something "bad".

This is the piece that remains hidden; we are susceptible to this programming to feel badly about ourselves and fearful about our food choices, and often we don't even know it. Instead of being seen as something that nourishes and sustains us, food becomes the enemy conspiring to make us fat.

My journey to weight loss was twofold. First I gave up dieting and all diet foods, and made peace with food. Then I changed my focus from weight loss to health.

The first step involved changing my thoughts and beliefs around food, diet, and body image. The second step, for me, involved juice cleansing to get my body nourished, and adopting an eating plan of whole, nutrient-dense food.

Do I ever stray from my healthy eating plan and eat something crappy? Hell yes! I am human. But I refuse to feel guilty about it. To the diet industry's chagrin, I eat whatever food it happens to be and enjoy it, rather than eat it and feel so guilty I get no pleasure from it, and overeat because I believed it was "bad" to eat it in the first place so I should never eat it again.

So there, take that, insane diet industry! There is another way—a peaceful way that won't leave you in the 68.5% overweight category.

Eat good food; feel good about what you eat.

This statement is the succinct version of my philosophy about what it takes to get back to your optimal weight and good health.

Eat good food. Here I use "good" not as my own personal label. By good I mean food that is whole and closest to its natural state. Food that is not modified; food that has nothing added or taken away. Food that is nutrient dense. Food that is not artificial.

In my coaching practice I invite people to find their own healthy eating style. One thing that I have concluded after three decades of dieting—there is no one "right" way to eat. If there were I wouldn't be writing this book. Each one of us is unique in our humanness, with unique bodily systems and belief systems. Your own healthy eating style needs to fit with both of these systems.

Some people thrive on a vegan plan, whether it is because of how they digest certain foods, their beliefs about ingesting animal protein and products, or both. Some do better with a version of what's referred to as the paleo or primal style, perhaps having some trouble digesting grains and legumes.

Some thrive on a diverse style, tolerating animal protein, grains, and dairy.

Feel good about what you eat. This, dare I say, is even more important than "eat good food". If you don't feel good about the food you are eating—whether it's a cookie or a carrot—you are going to be experiencing stress.

We hear about the hazards of stress all the time, but I don't know that we really heed the warnings. We are so conditioned to lead stressed-out lives that it feels normal. And we are super conditioned to feel stress when it comes to food.

This all stems from the "good" and "bad" labels we have learned to constantly place on ourselves and food. When we eat something we have learned to label "bad", we then, in turn, label ourselves as bad for eating it. I don't know how many times I have heard these words uttered by other people (and myself!) over the years, "I'm being bad today; the diet starts tomorrow," or, "I can't decide whether to be good or bad for lunch." How about this classic attitude, "Fuck it, I've been so bad this week I think I'll just eat the rest of this box of cookies"?

There is so much fear and self-loathing wrapped up in these statements I hardly know where to begin. We are treating ourselves as though we've committed a disgraceful crime when we eat something we consider bad, or more precisely that we think will make us gain weight. The bad label rarely implies bad for your health. No, "bad" means, *It will make me fat!* So if we ingest one of these bad foods, it makes us a bad person.

Wow, that's a lot of pressure. And a boatload of stress.

Science now shows us that much of what makes us gain weight is the tremendous stress we place on ourselves over what we are eating. The stress response causes what is known as a fight or flight reaction. We have become conditioned to view these "bad" foods as a danger. What happens when we encounter danger? We have to either fight off a predator or flee the situation.

This causes a physical response in the body. Blood flow is directed to the limbs, causing digestion to basically shut down. If you are running for your life your body's top priority is no longer digesting the burrito you had for lunch. This leads to digestive issues and food not getting assimilated properly. When you are not assimilating food properly you are not getting the nutrients you need, and you will soon be looking for something else to eat.

Another layer to this labeling disaster is that our thoughts get reflected back to us as our reality. Quantum physics tells us that, although we appear to be solid, at the subatomic level the smallest particles that make us up are actually waves of energy that can collapse into matter with intention. We are, as is everything, energetic, vibrational beings at our core. We are always offering a vibration, and our vibration attracts other like vibrations—once again, the good old law of attraction.

When we consistently feel like bad people because of our food choices, weight, or both, we are offering a low, fearful vibration. That fearful vibration is our point of attraction. From this point we are not focusing our thoughts on what we actually want, which is to be lean and healthy. We are instead focusing on the opposite: that we are not the size we want to be, that we are overweight, that we are bad. The reality we are creating is one that we are not going to like very much.

Having this unconscious focus on what we don't want is truly what trips people up when it comes to weight loss. Our thoughts and beliefs create our reality. Most of us have so many negative conditioned thoughts and beliefs around food, diet, and body image that we keep creating a reality we don't want. And then we blame ourselves for it.

You can see the cycle that is created here. When we don't feel good about what we are eating, no matter what it is, we are setting ourselves up for weight gain. Then we blame ourselves, beat ourselves up, and wonder why we never seem to be able to lose any weight. We have the day-to-day stressor of labeling ourselves and what we are eating as "bad" and hold an impossibly high standard of "good". Then we have the compounded stressor of being heavier than we deem acceptable, with our weight continuing to creep higher.

This leads to an acute unacceptance of ourselves. Before anything can shift in our outer reality, a big shift needs to happen on the inside. We must accept ourselves exactly as we are in every moment. We must move out of the low vibration of disdain toward ourselves and our bodies, and move into a vibration of acceptance and love. It's a tall order, I know, but this is the vibration from which we can return to our optimal weight and good health.

I encourage you to find a healthy eating style that you love and that feels best for you physically and emotionally. But this is just a guideline, and there will be many times when what you eat will fall outside of the plan you have adopted. When this happens, the most important thing you can do to stay on track and maintain your high vibration is to thoroughly enjoy what you are eating. Savor it; ooh and ah over it; delight in it. And when you are done eating, forget about it. There are a million better places to put your focus than on what you just ate. Drop the judgment; drop the labels. Feel **good** about what you ate.

As an example, shortly after I got back to my optimal weight, I went to a friend's house for a cookout. Some neighbors whom I hadn't yet met were there, and to my delight I ended up talking to one of them about drinking fresh pressed vegetable juices—my favorite subject! After finishing our conversation, I put my glass of (fermented grape) juice down and served myself one of Mark's perfectly grilled burgers. While I was obviously enjoying the hell out of it, the man came up to me, and with a little disgust in his voice said, "You do all this juicing, but now you are drinking wine and eating a burger?"

He was slapping the "bad" labels all over me. In the past this would have sent me reeling into shame and then desperately trying to explain myself for committing this terrible sin. Instead, with my newfound freedom of feeling good about whatever I ate, I simply said with great gusto, "Yes!"

The truth is that even before I lost the weight (in fact when I was at my heaviest) I had this phrase in my head: Eat good food; feel good about what you eat. I knew it was the key, even though I didn't know exactly how it was going to play out. Feeling good about whatever I ate put me in the vibrational space to allow the good food—the healthy eating plan that was perfect for me—to easily find me. I loved the way I was eating, and I didn't have the rigidity around it that had always accompanied a diet. I was just eating and enjoying whatever I was eating until I was done, and then I moved on to something else. Phew. What a relief.

Chapter 3

You Have to Accept It

When you try to force something, it usually breaks.

When I am in the process of making a big batch of juice, I sometimes try to get away with getting it all done without cleaning out the accumulated pulp midway. I end up trying to force the last few vegetables through the chute because there is too much pulp in the machine. You know what happens? It backs up. No matter how hard I push the vegetables they won't go through.

The backup is a clear sign that what I am doing isn't working. If I continue shoving vegetables down the shoot anyway you know what will happen next? The juicer will break.

What's the better choice—to continue to try to force it and be left with no way to make juice, or to take the time to clean it out and let the machine work the way it should, giving me juice for years to come? Logically, I would have to pick the latter.

Whenever I have tried to force anything in my life it has never worked. Trying to lose weight is a great example of this. For years and years I tried to force my body to become thin by going on all sorts of crazy diets that I didn't enjoy. I labeled foods as good or bad and judged them and myself against some diet model that somebody else made up. I forced myself to do something that I didn't want to be doing, and each time I eventually broke.

I broke. I couldn't sustain it. It wasn't natural, organic. It felt dreadful, which was a clear sign that it was not working. But I never heeded this sign—I just continued to try to force it until I broke.

After breaking over and over again, I finally got to the point where the pain of feeling so broken surpassed the pain of being overweight. I finally came to the place where I had to accept the fact that I was heavy, and that wasn't going to change overnight. After I found that acceptance, I knew in my heart that somehow the weight was going to come off naturally, in a way that wouldn't feel like a hardship.

That shift into acceptance alone made an immense difference in my life. While it took a little time to drop completely into it, my worry and judgment about food and my weight fell away. I felt a sense of peace, which I now realize was a clear sign that what I was doing *was* working, even though I didn't appear to be doing anything. Feeling that sense of peace got me into vibrational alignment so the right solution would appear. And low and behold, it did!

Weight loss is one example of something I tried unsuccessfully to force, but I see this phenomenon in every area of my life. Whenever I have tried to force anything—quitting smoking, exercise, relationships, business ventures, even finding a connection to my higher self—it has never worked out. The wonderful thing is that the breakdown always set me up to get to a better feeling place so I was able to allow the solution or the next best path to appear. The recognition of this has afforded me the opportunity to bypass the forcing/breaking step, and ease into acceptance in all areas of my life.

******

I think one of the hardest things for anyone to do is accept their body exactly the way it is. In my life I have run the gamut from being underweight to obese, but even when the scale was at the lowest I still had difficulty accepting my body. I was so conditioned to be at war with it, and in my mind I never met the standards I saw in the magazines and on TV.

This non-acceptance of ourselves is really a sad state of affairs. We are, in essence, rejecting ourselves. I'm sure we all have been in a situation of being rejected—whether it be by a lover, a business partner, a company for a potential job, or even a friend. It feels awful. It is a pain that can run very deep.

Yet on a daily basis many of us are rejecting our very selves. We wish for parts of our bodies to just go away. We berate ourselves first thing in the morning when we see the number on the scale. We continue this throughout the day, while getting dressed and, of course, while ingesting every morsel of food. Exercise, or lack of it, often comes into play; whether or not we were able to run the mileage we expected we should or how long we were able to hold that yoga pose. God forbid if we haven't been exercising at all—*what a slug!*

Imagine if someone else was saying the things to you that you were thinking all day long. Imagine your best friend looking over your shoulder at the number on the scale and saying, "WOW! You better get on that diet today! I don't know why you didn't start months ago." Or imagine a complete stranger yelling to you as you are walking down the street, "Oh my God—you look so FAT in those pants! Why on earth did you ever leave the house in them? You are huge!"

I would want to die if I heard those words coming from someone else. It is so incredibly hurtful. Yet for many of us, this negative self-talk is a constant dialogue in our heads. We say things to ourselves, and even aloud to others, that we would never say to another person—it would be far too mean. But we think talking to ourselves this way is fine, natural even. And we think it is natural when others say such things aloud about themselves.

We humans seem to have an endless array of things to worry and second guess ourselves about. But rejecting our body, this sacred vessel that we chose to incarnate in, every minute of every day, hating our very being—it is an atrocity!

It's as if we are waging a war against ourselves every day. Imagine the effect of that. It needs to stop, and it needs to stop right now. The good news is all it takes to stop this war is you!

******

How much time do you spend thinking about other people's feelings, worrying about whether you did something hurtful or that you haven't done enough? You may spend a fair amount of time doing that. Now it's time to start extending that courtesy to yourself.

How did we learn this horrid way of treating ourselves in the first place? Probably in a variety of ways—from our parents, our siblings, our friends, and, of course, the relentless diet industry. Berating ourselves, especially when it comes to diet and our bodies, is commonplace, and it is widely accepted. If we were acting this way toward another human it would be considered bullying—there is a no tolerance rule against that in schools. But treating ourselves in this way? The consensus is, *have at it! It would be strange if you didn't.*

It seems being kind to ourselves should be easy. We can be nice to everyone else—how hard can it be to treat ourselves in the same way? Well, as you likely know, it can be quite a challenge. But I cannot find strong enough words to impart the importance of taking on this challenge. In fact, I consider it fighting for your life.

******

As I've said, it took me a very long time to come to the understanding that I just had to accept what was true in the moment—that I was overweight and it wasn't going to change in an instant. It took a long time for the notion to occur to me that something big needed to change, and it wasn't my size. I had to change my attitude toward myself in a momentous way. It took so long for this seemingly obvious thing to compute because it wasn't obvious to me at all. Treating myself terribly was familiar and known, and, frankly, it helped me to fit in. Everybody was doing it—why wouldn't I?

I don't want you to wait another minute to take this step. Once I finally took the leap and committed to being kind and accepting of myself, the freedom I found was astounding.

Most of us believe that accepting ourselves as we are is like waving the white flag. Surrendering to what is means it will always be—that we are just giving up.

Nothing could be farther from the truth. The truth is we have to accept where we are in the moment for anything to be able to change. If we keep pushing against the thing we don't want, we are going to get more of it. Not accepting what is in this moment causes anger and fear to well up, so it is from anger and fear that we are creating our next moment. If we are creating our future from a place of fear, it's not going to turn out the way we want it to.

There is a tremendous feeling of freedom when we realize there is another way. And it is not just about weight loss— this realization effects our entire lives. When we accept what is, we start living from a place that is not filled with fear and anger. We learn to live from a place of love, because love and acceptance go hand in hand. A calm peace takes over. The war comes to an end.

******

I hope you are excited right now because there is some work involved. Self-acceptance is something that you will likely have to learn, as you are probably not used to being kind to yourself. But self-acceptance is like anything else—you must practice until it becomes a habit.

The first thing that has to shift is your concern about what other people are thinking. When I was heavy, I made comments about my size all the time so other people would know that I was well aware of how big I was. I wanted to make sure everyone knew that I knew I was fat; that I wasn't deluding myself by somehow thinking it was OK to be as large as I was. In my constant rejection of myself, I figured everyone else was going to reject me too. Better to let them know that I was aware of the situation and that I was trying to do something about it, right?

After I lost weight and was including before and after photos in my blog posts, it was wonderful to hear a few people say, "I never saw you as overweight. You were just Gwen." The truth is we don't know what other people are thinking, and whatever they are thinking is irrelevant. The only thing that matters is what we think, and that what we think about ourselves is positive and uplifting.

It is amazing to me how deep-seated our non-acceptance can be. In all my years of losing and gaining weight I was never happy with myself even when I was super thin. I have heard so many others say the same thing. "I've never been happy with my body."

I had an interesting experience after I got to the weight that felt right to me—people started calling me skinny. It was said in a not particularly nice way, as if they were happy for me but with a hint of disdain. I was referred to as, "That stick of a thing." I was told my legs were too thin. While shopping for new jeans I heard my good friend, who was acting as my personal shopper, discussing the problem that I had no ass with the sales guy!

These comments caused me to take a few steps back. I once again worried about what other people were thinking, and again wondered if I was OK the way I was. Although I was in the best shape of my life from running, I didn't have a whole lot of muscle tone. I thought, *That must be the problem!* I ran right out and hired a personal trainer and began lifting weights.

I gained some muscle tone, and in my quest not to have "too skinny legs" I put on a little weight. It was then I realized I had been happy at the weight I was—I felt the best at that size. I didn't stay true to my own good feelings about myself because I was worried about what other people were thinking. I was worried that once again I was unacceptable as I was. In reality, I had no way of knowing how people actually meant the things they said, nor should I have cared.

I defaulted to my old reaction, and put the unacceptable label on all by myself.

This non-acceptance is maddening and it is entirely bullshit! When will it end? The answer is it won't at some future time. You are not going to suddenly accept yourself when you hit a certain number on the scale, or a certain size of pants. This rejection of yourself has to end right now, in this moment, at whatever size you currently are.

If you don't accept yourself now, I think you can see how this is going to go—the thing you think will make you happy (weight loss or whatever it might be), and allow you to finally be kind to yourself, is never going to happen. Acceptance and kindness have to come first—they absolutely have to.

******

It is not really my way to tell other people what to do. I am all about, *There is no one right way to do anything.* As a coach, my intention is to help others find what works best for them, for example find their own healthy eating style. But there is no getting around this one—to lose excess weight or regain good health you absolutely have to do this: Accept where you are right now.

When I first started working with my business coach, on our very first call together he suggested that I go to Toastmasters to learn how to speak publically. I can hardly begin to express my distress at hearing this. My response was simulating the sound of throwing up. He asked, "What's the resistance?" I launched into a lengthy story about why it would be impossible for me to get up and speak in front of people, citing a presentation I had to give in college where I was shaking and nearly passed out—like an out of body experience, but not in a good way. Finally, I think just to shut me up, he said, "Well, you don't *have to*."

Of course, I was delighted with that news and we ended the call. I did, however, check out the Toastmasters website, just in case he brought it up again. I still had no intention of actually going.

On our next call together, one of the first things out of his mouth was, "What about Toastmasters—did you find a group?" I mumbled something about going to the website, but admitted I hadn't contacted anyone yet. Then he proceeded to badger me. "Why? You have to learn how to public speak—it would be so good for you! What are you going to do, sit in your house and write your blog all day? That's a nightmare!"

I started to panic, thinking, *How am I going to get out of this?* So, in the spirit of a true five-year-old, I raised my voice a little and said, "You said I didn't have to." His response to this, much as you would respond to a five-year-old, was, "Well, now you have to."

So I did go to Toastmasters, and it helped me tremendously in getting over my fear of public speaking, which changed my life in some amazing ways. But the point is I am always taken aback at the resistance we all have to the simple act of accepting ourselves.

No matter where your resistance level is, no matter how much you believe that beating yourself up is the way to weight loss and health, no matter what you say about why you can't accept yourself as you are right now, I can only say, "Well, now you have to." And, truly, you will be so glad you did!

******

So how do you go about this acceptance thing? I've said you have to, so now I should tell you how to do it, right? I can tell you that you're a divine being and absolutely perfect just the way you are, which is the complete truth. But nothing is going to change until *you* make a conscious decision to be kind to yourself, and stick to it in the very best way that you can.

There are great processes and methods to help change limiting thoughts and beliefs, some of which I use in my coaching practice. But, truthfully, when I made this shift to accepting myself, I didn't really use any of the many tools in my ever-growing tool box. Frankly, I was so tired of feeling shitty about myself that I just made the decision to stop. Then I remained vigilant—whenever I began to think or say something awful about myself, I caught it and stopped. I stopped the thought, or the sentence I had started to utter.

I did this over and over again until I trained myself out of the habit of negative self-talk. And, slowly but surely, I put more of my focus on things that I liked about myself, and all the good things that were currently in my life. I was proud of myself for going to Toastmasters, even though I still sucked at public speaking. I focused on what was working—*I'm going to Toastmasters!*—rather than what I perceived was not working—*I suck at public speaking!* And you can do that too!

To take on the challenge of accepting yourself right here in this moment is an amazing triumph. Some people will never come to this place, or even know it is an option. It becomes engrained in most of us pretty early on to be hard on ourselves. This new way is uncharted territory!

But it will be the most rewarding trek you will ever take, because once you find acceptance for yourself, you will be better able to accept whatever the moment brings. And that is where you find peace. I love living from this place. Please, please, join me!

Chapter 4

It's All Inside of You

I love the Buddha's attitude—essentially, it was, don't take what I'm saying as truth just because I'm saying it. Examine these teachings and take what resonates with you.

I've found there are parallels between spiritual seeking and dieting. It is great to research different paths. But when you look solely to one person or one philosophy to tell you what to do, that's when trouble starts to set in.

Why are there so many different diets, and so many different spiritual paths, if there is only one right way for everyone? Any diet book you pick up is going to prove beyond a shadow of a doubt that their plan is the only way to weight loss and health. Many religions tout that theirs is the only path to God. So, basically, if we don't choose right we are going to end up in a hell full of overweight, unhealthy people. That's a lot of pressure!

During my practically lifelong quest to lose weight, I finally found I had to give up dieting to have any chance of sanity and perhaps happiness. I had to give up my search for the Holy Grail—someone who could tell me how to eat so I would be thin. It was a desperate search but one I was much attached to. The solution had to be *out there* somewhere. It never occurred to me to look within; to look at what foods I felt the best eating.

******

For so many years I believed that there was one "right way" to eat to get to the "perfect" weight. I believed it was either out there and I hadn't found it yet, or that I had already found it, tried it, and failed at it. So I was on a constant quest to find a new diet, and if there was nothing new on the market I would go back to one of the diets I had already tried, thinking, *It will work this time if I don't screw it up.*

Like many of us, my relationship with food mirrored my relationship with life. I was convinced that somebody else had to tell me the right way to eat. I didn't even consider that maybe the "right" way to eat was inside of me; that I could tune in and listen to what my body wanted and needed. Nor did I consider that this "right" way might change over time.

When I was a senior in high school trying to figure out what my college major would be I knew I wanted to study something like psychology or social work—that was where my heart was drawn. My mom thought I was too sensitive to do social work—it would be too upsetting for me. My guidance counselor said, "You won't make enough money doing social work. You should major in business."

The next thing I knew I was applying to UMass Amherst Business School. Shortly after that, there I was enrolled with a full boat of business classes … that I hated.

I chose psychology or sociology for all my electives. I was excited about these classes and decided to minor in sociology. I also took a writing course, which I loved and did well in. But it never occurred to me to change my major. I was told to major in business—why would I consider pursuing a major that made me happy?

What was I thinking? I hated the business classes—what did I think working in the field was going to be like? I had no idea what I would even do with a business degree; I couldn't even picture what kind of a job I would get. But I knew it was the right thing to do, because that's what I was told.

No wonder I was so depressed in college! I did manage to graduate after taking some time off. (A good friend finally told my parents I was losing it and shouldn't be in school.) I took a year off, waitressed, and got into a bad relationship. What I didn't do was give any thought to what I might like to be doing. Then I went back and finished my business degree.

After graduation, my mom bought me a suit to wear to all my job interviews. I never wore that suit once. I went right back to my waitressing job (which I hated as well) and continued on in my bad relationship. Once again, I didn't give any thought to what I might like to be doing, what might feed my soul. Oh, and I ramped up my dieting after said boyfriend told me I was too heavy.

With food, and with the rest of my life, I constantly sought out other people to tell me what I should do, and their opinions rarely ended up pointing me toward things that were joyful to me. But I continued to do them anyway, while slowly self-destructing in my spare time.

I became a nervous wreck and an awesome dieter. Back in my twenties I could sustain a crazy awful diet long enough to lose a bunch of weight. Armed with the news that I was too heavy, my life's purpose became to be super thin. And lose weight I did, to the point where this same awesome boyfriend informed me one day when I sat on his lap that I had lost too much weight and my ass was too boney. I still wasn't good enough.

Never once in all this time did I ever consider myself. What did I like to do? What did I like to eat? What foods made me feel the best? What type of exercise did I like to do?

I didn't have any hobbies, unless you count drinking wine. I simply spent my life trying to maintain—maintain my terrible relationship, maintain my stressful job, maintain my weight, and maintain my continuously fraying nerves. I hated myself and I hated my life.

In hindsight, feeling this way was actually fantastic because it brought me a huge gift. It caused me to start seeking. I was so miserable, so sad, such a wreck, and I started to wonder, *Why the hell am I here? Do we really just come into this world, live an awful life, and then die?* It didn't make any sense—I needed to find out more.

Around this time my general anxiety increased to full out panic. Luckily, I never had a panic attack at work so I was able to keep my job. But other than that, leaving my house was a nightmare. My world became very small and completely filled with fear. I knew something had to change, but I had no idea how to change anything, so I started to read.

Finally, I had a hobby, even though I didn't actually realize it. My hobby was seeking my higher self and finding a whole new way to live.

******

Now I can see that becoming an emotional wreck was the best thing that could have happened to me. If I hadn't been so miserable, so distraught, I might not have ever been curious about whether there was something more to life. I might have just schlepped along in my mediocre existence, simply maintaining. Instead, I began to open up to a richness of life that I hadn't ever experienced. And it was this richness that many years later helped me to shift my relationship with food and weight.

I read everything I could get my hands on about spirituality, near death experiences, what happens after we die, and later on everything about how we manifest things into our lives. I went to different mediums and psychics and had readings. I became interested in energy work and studied Reiki and Healing Touch. I spent a month at Kripalu Center for Yoga and Health earning a Holistic Health Teacher Training certificate. I got certified in Neuro Linguistic Programing, and studied Emotional Freedom Techniques.

I was actually doing things that I liked … as a hobby. I started to write. I decided I was going to write a book that I called *From Depression Into Being*, subtitled *An Ordinary Woman's Journey*. I figured there were plenty of famous people out there writing about their journeys through tough times—why couldn't I? I decided I was going to write myself out of this dark place I was still largely living in, so I would not only end up with a book but that book would have a triumphant ending I didn't even know about yet! I didn't realize that the final piece would be changing my relationship with food and diet.

I never did finish that book. I recently pulled it out to see where I had stopped writing—I stopped writing right as I stopped dieting. I didn't consciously stop writing. I think the liberation of quitting dieting catapulted me over the hurdle from depression into being. It's like I chronicled it without chronicling it—I said it without saying it at all. I didn't need to write about it—I just needed to live it; to be with it and see where it would take me. And where it took me birthed a whole new book—the very book you are reading.

I wrote the last few paragraphs of *From Depression Into Being* after returning home from a trip to Belize. I was at my heaviest but being out of the country made me feel better about myself. There were women of all shapes and sizes, and no one was talking about the diet they needed to go on or lamenting the piece of bread they just ate. There seemed to be a general acceptance of differing body size, rather than judgment.

Then, one night, while out at a dance club, I heard the nicest thing anyone has ever said to me. While waiting for my friend Chuck to retrieve drinks at the busy bar, a handsome, young Belizean man walked up to me, grabbed my hand, and said, "I like your size."

I wish someone had caught that moment on tape! I can only imagine how big my smile was as I gushed, "You do?" Someone was complimenting me on the thing that had continuously caused me the most angst for all of my adult life, and especially then, at my heaviest. This stranger was letting me know I was actually OK. I glanced over my shoulder to keep my eye on Chuck so I wouldn't lose him just as he was walking towards us—he tells me that I had *the look of love* on my face (and, of course, we found the whole incident hysterically funny, making great fodder for the rest of the trip and beyond).

The following is the last of what I wrote after I talked about the trip to Belize and my boyfriend of five minutes:

I made a decision. I made the decision to stop dieting. I was freaked out because I didn't want my weight to continue to go up. I remember at one point lamenting to a friend, "I'm worried about my skin—that it has stretched out too much." She replied, "Well, don't get any fatter." The real problem didn't hit me then—her statement just made me panic even more. But later, when I honestly thought about it, I knew that dieting, not eating, had made me this fat. I knew deep down that I had to stop it even though I was desperate to do the diet thing and lose weight. I knew I could lose weight—I had always been able to. But I had to face the reality that it ALWAYS CAME BACK. Not only the weight I lost, but MORE THAN I LOST CAME BACK. Every time. Period. I had wrecked myself. Now it was time to reverse the trend.

So I decided, a little reluctantly, to quit dieting. I was going to eat what I wanted when I wanted. I was going to try not to overeat but I was prepared to accept myself if I did. I started my process by eliminating diet foods, except the ones I didn't mind like light mayo or salad dressing. I did this for about a month when I realized I hadn't given up dieting at all. I was still eating diet foods. It was then that I completely renounced dieting, which was liberating beyond belief, and in some ways scary as hell.

One of my favorite things now is whole milk yogurt. Have you ever tried it? If you are like most people I've encountered, you have not. Yogurt is supposed to be a "healthy" food so you have to get the nonfat. I'm going to say this right now, and I think you all will agree, albeit secretly—eating nonfat yogurt is like eating nothing. No, it's worse than eating nothing because it gets your system fired up for more food, and of course you don't give it any since you were just having your light breakfast. I am hungry a second after I eat a nonfat yogurt. No, I take that back. I am hungry before I finish eating a nonfat yogurt. I want an omelet or something after, no during, eating a nonfat yogurt.

I persevered, and my weight stabilized. That was a huge hurdle for me. I ate real food. I tried the best that I could not to eat food that was overly processed, but on occasion I would grab an egg (egg product) and cheese (square of processed American) on a croissant (seems like a croissant) at Dunkin Donuts on my way out of town to drive across the state to see my dad. It's the only place that's convenient to stop, so it's OK. I don't get obsessed or bothered by it, feeling like I shouldn't be eating it. Basically, I eat what I feel like eating, and I give it some thought first.

******

Eighty-six pages single spaced I had written, and I just stopped. I see why now—making the decision to quit dieting was the beginning of my path to making peace with food. It was also when I really started listening to myself. I started taking myself into consideration—what did I like, what did I want? Doing this caused me to feel more peaceful—I no longer needed to "write myself" out of depression.

At first, my rant about the yogurt seemed a little excessive, but now I understand that too—because it used to freak people out when I ate it. *How can you eat that? It's* full *fat!* Friends who were not even overweight often made such comments because we are so strongly conditioned to think fat is "bad".

Times like those were uncomfortable, but it was all so worth it. I see now that, as I learned how to stay true to myself through my food choices and my approach to eating, I slowly began to remain true to myself in other areas of my life.

I learned how to say no. I had been, practically since birth, a relentless people pleaser. Fueled by a desperate fear of not being loved, I always said yes when friends or family asked me to do anything, even if I didn't want to. I felt that I had to say yes—if I didn't they might get angry with me, or, worse still, dump me out of their life. I couldn't chance it.

Once I realized I didn't want to eat in a way that made me miserable, I began to wonder, *Why do I do anything that makes me miserable?* I realized that my friends would understand if something didn't appeal to me or if there was something I would rather do than what they were suggesting. And they do, I think. I did ruffle some feathers though. People were so used to me agreeing with them that it was surprising, and a little off-putting, when I said no. But guess what—they are still my friends. And I am a much happier person.

This shift in me also affected my work life. For so many years I had worked at jobs I didn't like. When I got laid off from my position at a mortgage company, I finally worked up the courage to strike out on my own and utilize all of the trainings I had taken.

I worked with people one-on-one and began writing a blog. Writing called to me the most but I felt as though I "should" be putting most of my efforts into coaching.

Luckily, the Universe stepped in. I wasn't getting consistent coaching clients. It was a struggle. Finally, I realized, *I shouldn't be doing this right now if it feels like a struggle. I'm not enjoying it so it is not going to flow.*

I love to write. After I began to put more of my focus there I was asked to write a book. Although that opportunity didn't work out, it opened up other doors leading to me writing this book. All because I stayed true to myself and what I wanted—I stayed in the flow.

Even when I think of all the other things I have to do to make it as a writer, which is overwhelming, I still want to do it. You know why? Because it feels good, and when you are doing what feels good you are simply going with the current rather than trying to swim against it. You are flowing with your own high vibration, and it carries you.

We are all unique—there is no one "right" way for anything. So with food, and with life, it is time to stop looking out there for a solution, and go within. It's all inside of you.

Chapter 5

Dumping the Diet Mentality

So, I've talked a little bit about the law of attraction—that we are all vibrational beings at our core, and that like vibration attracts like vibration. You may already be familiar with this concept and adept at attracting certain things into your life. Perhaps you always get the best parking spot in a crowded lot.

But does this notion seem to fail you when it comes to weight loss? Or do you think it doesn't even apply?

Well, I must tell you that the law of attraction never fails you and, yes, it applies to everything.

So why can't you lose the weight? Should be easy, right?

Yes—RIGHT! Believe it or not, it can be easy but you have to radically change your thoughts and beliefs to attract what it is you *want*, which is weight loss, instead of focusing on what you don't want, lack of weight loss.

Many of us have a conditioned belief that we are not good enough—that our bodies are simply unacceptable. The solution we are given to fix this problem is to diet. *Have some willpower for God's sake!*

Yet in the US, as a nation we are getting heavier and heavier. What is wrong here?

Pretty much everything.

First of all, you must believe, no matter what you weigh, that THERE IS NOTHING WRONG WITH YOU! Your weight or size is not who you are. It is just the most current manifestation of your physical form.

After my mom died I was home trying to help my dad out. I can't even recall how it came up but he told me he would pay me to lose weight—10 bucks a pound. Then he proceeded to explain, "Say, if you lose 100 pounds you would get 1000 dollars."

OK, I was pretty overweight. Regardless, to hear that was shocking, and it made me realize how my own father saw me—100 or more pounds overweight—and he thought offering to pay me would be an incentive, like I wouldn't care about losing the weight otherwise.

I'm sure his intention behind this offer was well meaning. He probably was seeing this woman, his daughter, who would likely never marry and have a family because she was fat.

I laughed it off, saying, "100 pounds?" Even my brother, who will gladly take any opportunity to make fun of me, said, "Yeah, Jesus dad, 100 pounds?" My dad laughed and said something about he was just doing the calculation. Too late—it was already burned into my brain.

But here's my point: we are constantly bombarded by the "fact" that we are not good enough as we are, sometimes even from the people closest to us.

And that leads to the law of attraction *failing us*. Oh, wait, that never happens.

What does happen is that our thoughts and beliefs about ourselves and our ideas about how to fix the problem of not being good enough are totally out of whack. Instead of solving anything, they are actually perpetuating the perceived problem.

Until we change these thoughts and beliefs we are going to keep getting the same results. We might be able to force the weight off for a period of time, but if we continue to believe that we are still not good enough, it will come back.

If you are struggling with weight, please know THERE IS NOTHING WRONG WITH YOU! That is just what you have been led to believe. And that belief can be changed.

******

A belief is just a thought you think over and over again until it becomes a truth for you. Our beliefs about ourselves and the world begin to form when we are quite young. Unfortunately, we don't have much of a say in what beliefs we end up with—they are a product of conditioning by our parents, siblings, peers, mentors, and society. These conditioned beliefs can cause problems in many aspects of our lives, but when it comes to food, eating, and body image they can really wreak havoc!

From a young age I learned from advertisements, television, and the general culture that it was important to be thin, and beautiful.

Initially, weight wasn't something I considered to be problematic. My mom was thin and there weren't any food restrictions in our house. But then my mom developed a thyroid condition and put on a bunch of weight. As a result, dieting became a way of life for her.

This is when I started to get conditioned to eat diet "foods" rather than whole food. Light this and low-fat/non-fat that became regular items in our house. And always artificial sweeteners. I am not saying this to place blame—it is what we were told to do at the time to lose weight and be healthy. Now there is a lot of information available about the perils of eating this way, and that it can actually cause weight gain. Yet there are still hordes of people who subscribe to it. Why? Because they were conditioned to *believe* that it is the *right* way to eat to lose weight.

My introduction to dieting came at the same time that I was going into junior high, and although I hadn't before considered that I had a weight problem, I felt anything but beautiful. I learned and believed that beauty was an important criterion in order for me to fit in and have friends. I couldn't do anything about my big nose and glasses, but I could lose some weight—it seemed like the right thing to do.

You can probably see that the above decision made absolutely no sense. I was thin—one thing I had going for me. But my belief that I wasn't good enough, that I didn't fit the standards of society, on top of seeing my mom constantly on a diet, informed this brilliant decision—a decision that caused me a lot of suffering for the next thirty or so years.

It is amazing to me how we operate as humans. We will continue to repeat patterns over and over and over again, seeing each time that it didn't work out, because we believe it is the right way.

This sounds kind of sad, like we have this robotic quality, doing what has been programed into us. While in a sense this is true, it also holds the greatest hope and promise. Unlike robots, we have the capacity to change our thoughts and beliefs; we have the capacity to enter a new program.

That is great news, wouldn't you say? It sounds so simple! And it is. The only tricky thing is we don't really want to.

Sounds crazy—why wouldn't I want to change a belief that clearly isn't serving me? The answer is because it's familiar.

Our thoughts and beliefs evoke emotions. An emotion causes chemical events to occur in our body. Regardless of whether these chemical events cause a pleasant feeling or an unpleasant feeling, when it happens over and over again our body becomes accustomed to it. It becomes a familiar feeling and we look to recreate it.

Beliefs that are formed at a young age have been kicking around in our systems for a long time. That means we have been feeling the same feelings for a long time. The feelings are very familiar to us, which makes them comforting even when they are unpleasant.

Even though I got to the point, probably in my thirties, where I could see clearly and intellectually that dieting wasn't working, in fact that it was causing me to gain more weight, I had a very hard time letting it go. I believed so much in being on a diet, that it was the only way to get back to my thin self, that I continued my desperate search for the latest fad despite having this knowledge.

Right here I think we can see the huge conundrum anyone struggling with weight faces. We have such strong beliefs in how weight loss is supposed to go, and also about how we are supposed to look, that even when presented with another way, we resist it.

******

Two things had to happen in order for me to lose the weight for good. As I talked about earlier, I had to truly accept myself where I was in the moment. The second thing was I had to radically change my thoughts and beliefs around food, diet, and body image. I finally realized I was going to have to train myself not to be on a diet; train myself to stop thinking about it and talking about it; train myself to just eat without all the judgment.

It is funny to write this because you would think that this would be any dieter's dream come true—to just be able to eat. But, again, we are used to all the strict rules we have set for ourselves based on our belief in dieting. Just eating is so unfamiliar, so unknown, it almost feels undoable.

I remember the relief I felt when I made the decision that, yes, I was going to quit dieting! It did seem like a dream come true ... and then too good to be true. The excitement of being able to eat whatever I wanted whenever I wanted would quickly turn into fear. I couldn't even recall what it was like because it had been so long since I had simply eaten. *This can't be right. I'd better find a new diet.*

Aside from the familiar feeling there was also that rush of adrenaline when starting a new diet. There was that tremendous hope of a new life—a thin life where everything always worked out. But I never thought about the fact that, even if I lost weight, I would still have the same awful job, the same anxious thoughts, and perhaps, maybe, I would meet a guy who liked me but the relationship would probably end up like all my others—crappy.

We get so stuck in these patterns that it's hard to see that we don't just have bad luck. We can't see that nothing is going to change in our lives until we change our thoughts and beliefs, including and especially around weight loss.

The good news here is that we can change our thoughts and beliefs and it is simple to do. Simple but not so easy. The conditioning we have runs deep. This means we have to literally train ourselves to think in a different way.

******

To illustrate this point—I haven't been exercising much lately, and I use the word much lightly. I finally decided this morning to at least get out for a walk.

As I was walking along, it became apparent that things are not as tight as they were just a month ago. It was also apparent that I am not in the shape I was last year, or even six months ago.

Normally this news would send me straight to the arsenal of mean things to say. I would walk along berating myself, generally feeling like a "bad" person for letting this happen.

On top of all that I would start to get this panicky feeling— *Suppose I start gaining weight! How have I let myself stop exercising this month? How am I going to get back in the shape I was? I have totally blown it!*

This chatter could easily send me directly to *fuck it* land; do not pass go, do not collect 200 dollars.

Instead, I looked out at the river where it spills into the ocean and thought, as I often do, about how beautiful Newburyport is. Walking along the waterfront is gorgeous. Walking the beach is amazing and one of my favorite things to do. I can just enjoy walking around until I start to get my feet back under me and can do a little running. Plus, I thought it would be fun to have a little challenge and it would give me an opportunity to clean up my eating a bit.

Same situation and two very different perceptions. Which one do you think is more helpful?

I was talking with a good friend a few days ago who has been thin and fit, I believe, all of her adult life. She certainly has as long as I have known her. She is beautiful inside and out. She said something like, "Intellectually, I know that I am not overweight and that I am in better shape than most women my age. But I'm walking around and I still feel like that fat five-year-old. I can still feel the way that feels—how uncomfortable it was, that heavy feeling. Sometimes I see a pair of my small sized pants and I think, *Whose are those? They certainly aren't mine.*"

No matter what size or shape we are, most of us are trained to do the same thing—to think about what is "wrong" with us, even if it was decades ago. We got conditioned early on to find fault with ourselves. We learned somewhere along the line that we were not good enough. So, instead of focusing on the things that we intellectually know are working in our lives, it feels more normal to focus on what we consider to be wrong with us.

I am so grateful for today and the different, useful chatter that was in my head. But I will tell you it didn't happen overnight. We absolutely can change our thoughts and beliefs so we can live more peaceful lives. Again, we have to train ourselves to do it.

There are awesome tools out there to help shift limiting beliefs, so we can speed up the process. But the first step is simple awareness—being aware of the thoughts we are thinking and when they are unhelpful, or should I say mean, stopping right there in the moment. Stop mid-sentence if you are saying it aloud. You can replace it with a more helpful thought but the most important thing is to just stop it. Keep doing this over and over again, and after a while you will form a new habit of thinking. And that habit of thinking will likely spill over into other areas of your life.

For me, making peace with food—and, in the process, thinking different thoughts about myself—opened a door. Now being kind to myself feels generally normal so I am able to do it in other areas of my life. I have found a level of peace I once thought was impossible. Changing my relationship with food, and, in turn, with myself, opened that door for me.

If you often go to the arsenal of mean things to say when it comes to food, diet, or body image, please consider opening this door yourself. Believe me, you will be beyond happy that you did.

******

The diet mentality has so much wrapped up in it. Changing how we think and talk about ourselves is huge and will prove to be the biggest hurdle for many, again, as this conditioning runs so deep. The next piece of this puzzle that must be addressed is labeling and judging food, and ourselves, as "good" or "bad".

How many times have you said, "I'm being good today so I'll just have a salad," or, while eating a muffin on vacation, "I'll be bad for the rest of the day because I'm on vacation but the diet starts tomorrow"?

On top of this labeling there is also the general diet talk that goes on constantly. "I just started on a low fat high carb diet. How about you?" "Oh, no, that doesn't work—I'm doing Atkins. It's the only way to go." "How come that skinny bitch over there can eat whatever she wants and never gains any weight?" Not to mention all the lamenting about having to be on a diet in the first place.

Imagine how much time you would have if you eliminated this topic from your conversations. Imagine how much more time you would have if you also eliminated this topic from your thoughts.

Wow—you would have time to write a book! At least that's what I have found. But, better yet, it is incredibly freeing once you have trained yourself to stop doing it. The judgments we place on ourselves and on the food we put into our mouths are so incredibly harsh. It is a huge relief when you stop it!

This, again, is something we are conditioned to do. You probably don't even notice it, particularly when one of your friends is talking "diet talk". Start to take note of it—you'll be amazed at how much you hear this talk from other people, even from that skinny bitch who you think has it made.

I have encountered people who don't seem to engage in this kind of conversation but, in my experience, they are not in the majority. When you start to shift away from everything diet related you will be bucking the cultural norm, which can be uncomfortable. But it truly is the key to getting back to your natural size, and, more exciting than that, it is the key to unlock the door to peaceful living.

******

The whole concept of dumping the diet mentality probably sounds pretty good to you right now, and simple enough to do. I will say it again; it is simple but it honestly is not easy. I say that not to discourage you but to empower you to stick with it.

This is the rest of your life we are talking about. How do you want to live it? Now is the time to make a CONSCIOUS DECISION to break out of this prison you have been living in. Now is the time to make this choice and then practice, practice, practice it until it becomes your new habit of thinking.

You may have some false starts; I know I did. It takes fortitude to forge your own path. It is our human nature to want things to stay the same, to stay familiar even when the familiar is painful.

Friends, family, co-workers—they are all used to the dieting you. They will want to engage with you in the same way they have always done. They will want to continue to bond over berating themselves about the cookie they just ate. It may feel like some sort of a betrayal to avoid engaging with them in this way anymore. So here is one more mindset to shift—pleasing other people.

Here is where you have to ask yourself, "Is sticking with the cultural norm, and making everyone else feel comfortable where they are stuck, worth staying stuck myself?"

I am writing this book so I can tell you—it absolutely is not worth it! Once you get through this bit of discomfort and your new habit solidifies, you will experience a level of freedom that you may never have known. I know I did. Dumping the diet mentality, thereby making peace with food and with myself, was the greatest gift I have ever given myself.

It truly is a gift and it is one that you can give to others simply by your own example. As I made my transition away from dieting it did make people in my life uncomfortable. It didn't fit into most of their belief systems. They didn't understand how I could *not* be on a diet.

But this critical step of dumping my diet mentality, of stopping the judgment and anxious stream of thoughts and words, put me into a new vibrational state where I was able to find what I needed to sustainably and easily lose the weight.

Going through this journey has given me the opportunity to share it with others, to share this huge gift of freedom I feel I have been given. As you shift into a peaceful place around food, diet, and body image, people in your life will see a new possibility. They will see that, despite their conditioning, there is another way.

They won't necessarily jump right on the bandwagon. But seeing your transition will cause a spark in them. You can be part of a new movement towards peace. What an amazing gift to give to yourself, and to the world!

Chapter 6

Food Should Not Be Frightening

The last quarter of this year I have spent a lot of time contemplating how we as a society and culture feel about food … and it's not good!

Food = Fear to many, many people. We are afraid of the thing that is meant to nourish us and that we need to survive!

We don't know what to eat; we are told so many different things by the experts in weight loss and nutrition and a lot of the information seems to contradict itself. Even me and my touting of green juice. I love juicing and it has changed my life and health profoundly. But some people just don't like it, while it will be fantastic for others. It all depends on your system and what health issues are going on. Smoothies might be a better choice for those who are trying to get in more vegetables.

I equate juicing with freedom. But I realize now that for many juicing incites fear. It is another thing that they "should" be doing, and quite frankly they don't want to. They are hugely resistant to it for whatever reason, right down to it is a pain to clean up. There is also fear of having it be just another diet that they can't stand to be on. There is fear of deprivation, even though a lot of the foods that they don't want to be deprived of are causing fear of weight gain.

OK, this is a pretty screwed up system! How can we win when both the perceived healthy and unhealthy foods are causing stress and angst? Where do you go from there?

It has become clear to me that if a food is causing you anxiety, you should not be ingesting it. Period. It is toxic—not because of the food but because of your thoughts about the food.

Think about it—how do your current beliefs about food and what you should or shouldn't be eating make you feel? I think for many people the answer is going to be, "Not good!"

We need to start a new food revolution—focused not on what we eat, but on how we feel about food!

Imagine if every time you ate it was a celebration, no matter what it was that you were putting in your mouth. Imagine if you sat down and tasted and savored your food. Imagine if you shut off the TV and had lovely, relaxed conversation while you enjoyed and paid attention to what you were eating, or just sat quietly. Imagine if you felt **peaceful** every time you ate.

******

Food should not be frightening. I can still recall the intense fear and panic I felt when my weight went up. Then every meal became a nightmare—the agony of trying to choose between the diet meal and what I really wanted to eat. Either choice would cause anxiety, with feelings of either deprivation or guilt.

There's no getting around it—we have to eat. And it's not just once in a while. We have to eat many, many times—many times a day even. Preparing food and eating can take up a good chunk of our day. Do we really want that time to be unpleasant?

Making peace with food goes hand in hand with dumping the diet mentality, and, of course, accepting ourselves where we are in the moment. But to me it is the most special, sacred part. Because when we are peaceful around food, we are truly nourishing ourselves.

Sure, I have adopted a healthy eating style that works best for me. For some reason I don't usually digest beans well, and grains often leave me feeling bloated. But if I am in a really relaxed setting with good friends enjoying a leisurely meal I will often eat these things and they will not bother me at all. Why? Because I am feeling good.

I am relaxed. I am enjoying the tastes of all the different foods. I am enjoying the conversation. Nobody is rushing. Nobody is talking about how they shouldn't be eating what they are eating. The only food talk is exclamations like, "This is amazingly delicious!" and the slight hum of, "Mmm mm mmmmmmmm MMMMM!" The food is being savored.

Yet I feel very differently when I am eating with folks who are not feeling peaceful with their food choices. If there is a lot of diet related talk or good and bad labeling, even though I am not joining in with this per se, it causes me to feel an underlying low level of stress. I could be eating the exact same meal, but this time I might end up overeating, and either way I will likely have a stomach ache later.

I am ingesting exactly the same thing. One time it doesn't cause any problem, the next time it does. The difference? Eating in peace or eating under stress.

I am going to take a guess here, but what do you think is the most common thing people do while eating? I'm sure you've guessed what I am going to say—watch television. What's playing on the TV? Possibly the news—ugh! What's more stressful than that? But even if you are watching something enjoyable or funny, chances are that you are not very aware of what you are eating, or even that you are eating.

It's funny when I think about it coming from my dieting background. When dieting, all I wanted to do was be able to eat. But then when I ate I would sit in front of the TV. I don't know why I would want to take anything away from eating, but, honestly, to just sit there by myself and eat seemed strange—I felt like I needed to be doing something else as well. Even when I lived with a partner we would still sit in front of the TV. OK, I suppose that says something about the relationship, but I wonder why I wouldn't want to enjoy a relaxed eating experience.

I think we often distract ourselves while eating because we don't feel like we deserve to be eating in the first place. Imagine that—we feel like we don't deserve to be nourished. Man, that makes me sad when I think about it—many of us feel like we don't deserve to get our most basic needs met. If you are amongst this group it is definitely time for that to shift!

******

Very simply, this once again takes practice. For many of us it is not a normal state to be relaxed around food. We may not even notice we are stressed so we must become keenly aware of our state of being when we sit down to eat. And we have to hang on to that awareness because even after we shift these old patterns they still can linger, and on occasion they will pop in to say hello.

When I spent time in Mexico at an all-inclusive place, my old patterns showed up as uninvited guests. I went from enjoying all the different foods to being freaked out that I was eating a lot of foods I didn't normally eat much of. I was trying to get my coaching practice going, which was mainly focused around weight loss. *What if I gain weight? I can't gain weight if I want to do this work!* I started to feel bloated and things weren't fitting right. Was this because of what I was eating … or what I was thinking? My stressed self wanted to tell me it was all about what I was eating, but my peaceful self knew the latter was really the truth.

Having a few blips like this from time to time actually makes me feel blessed, because I now know there is another way— that I can be peaceful around food and let it nourish me. I can enjoy what I am eating and then move on. Experiencing this peace, at my heaviest weight in fact, changed my entire life. Stopping dieting and being peaceful with food and eating removed my biggest stress. So even though I still had the desire to get back to my thin self, the desire came from a different place. It was no longer a fearful, panicked desire. It was a compassionate desire and I knew deep in my heart that it would happen just the way it was supposed to.

Awareness is really the key. Remember, this stressed feeling around food and eating likely feels normal to you so you may not even notice it. This means you have to consciously check in with yourself. When you go to have something to eat how are you feeling? Are you relaxed or tense? If you are feeling tense, stop and take a few deep breaths. Check in with your thoughts. If thoughts about how this food is going to make you fat and you are a bad person for eating it are running through your mind, those thoughts need to be flipped. *This food nourishes my body. I am going to enjoy eating something I love. I am giving my body the fuel it needs.*

I know this sounds simplistic, and it is because all you are doing is breaking a habit. You are breaking the pattern of your mind going directly to your negative thoughts that you are used to thinking. Come up with your own positive phrases that resonate and are believable to you. Take a few more deep breaths and then check in again—*Am I feeling relaxed about eating this food?* If the answer continues to be no, listen to your gut—*Is there something I would rather be eating right now?* Most likely the answer will be yes. It is really important to get into the habit of avoiding eating anything that is causing you stress.

We live in a fast paced culture where we have lost the sense of importance of taking time out for a meal. Many of us eat on the run, in our car, or while working at our desks. If we are at home there are other distractions—the TV, a magazine you wanted to flip through, or your children's homework. This habit of eating while doing something else is a big one for many of us. And it is time to break it.

Really, where is the joy of eating if we don't even know we are doing it? I would imagine some of you are feeling resistance to this as you are reading it. You may be thinking, *I don't have time to have breakfast at home—I have to eat on the way to work. I have too much work to do—I have to eat at my desk. I like eating dinner in front of the TV—it's relaxing.* If you live alone or eat many of your meals alone you might be thinking, *What—I'm supposed to just sit there by myself and eat?* Yes!

This was a big one for me. When I started to break this habit I did live alone and worked alone. My habit for dinner was eating in front of the Food Network. So I would be eating while watching somebody else cook something other than what I was eating.

That was pretty dumb. Eating is supposed to be a pleasing sensory experience. Instead of being focused on the yummy aromas or tastes of what I was eating, I was thinking about the tastes and aromas of the food on the television. Seems like that would kind of cancel out what I was actually eating.

When I decided to be committed to eating mindfully, it did seem very odd to me to sit down at the kitchen table with my plate of food, nary a book or magazine in sight, and just eat. I was so used to doing other things when I ate that it almost seemed foolish to *just* be sitting there eating. Now I've finally realized the foolish thing was me missing out on the pleasure of the food I was eating because I wasn't paying attention to it.

One more thing to take a look at—how fast are you eating? I am grateful that I have always been a slow eater so I haven't had to overcome this hurdle. As a matter of fact, I remember as far back as high school my friends would always finish eating lunch before me. They got bored waiting for me to finish so they would get up and take my tray away with the rest of my lunch still on it! If you can relate, always the first to finish your meal, this is another habit to work on breaking because the next piece to address is relearning our hungry and full signals.

******

We have learned to eat for so many reasons other than the simple fact that we are hungry. We eat because it is "time" for lunch, we eat because we are bored or because we are sad, or maybe because we are happy. That's OK and that is still going to happen from time to time. But it is a really powerful thing to get back in touch with our body's natural signals—what it feels like to feel hungry, and what it feels like to feel full.

I had the hungry part down—for so many years I was on so many diets and feeling hungry much of the time. But I wouldn't necessarily eat when I was hungry so my body likely started saying, "What the hell—is there some sort of famine going on?" Then when I would break down and eat something I would be ravenous. If it was something I had labeled as "bad" then I would not heed the full signal, feeling like I shouldn't be eating this food in the first place so I better eat a lot of it. I was either feeling hungry, or starving, and ignoring it, or I was overeating and feeling sick. Both of those scenarios pretty much suck.

And if you are a fast eater then I'm sure you have encountered becoming overly full because by the time you realized you were full, you had already eaten much more than you needed.

Again, what is called for here is awareness. It's time to start letting your body feel safe again by heeding its signals. Our bodies want and need to be nourished by the food we are eating—not to be left starving or to feel sick. We certainly wouldn't want that for someone else so why would we think that it's fine to treat ourselves this way?

There are a lot of facets to making peace with food. It takes changing some deep-seated habits and conditioning, and that's OK. All you have to do in this moment is have a willingness to explore the possibility. Just imagine having the sensation of hunger and taking that as a signal to feed yourself. Imagine checking in to determine what you feel like eating. Imagine sitting and eating that food with your total attention, savoring the experience, recognizing your full signal and stopping, feeling safe knowing that if you are hungry even five minutes later you can eat that food again. Imagine feeling relaxed and satisfied after every eating experience.

I want you to imagine it because it is likely not what your current reality looks like. You might feel like it's too much to change—is it really worth it? I am here to tell you that it is absolutely 100% worth it. Feeling peaceful while eating is such a wonderful experience. Just eating, without distraction, without judgment, is one of the best changes I have ever made. It has totally changed my life, and it can change yours too. You just have to be open to the possibility— it is possible to make peace with food, and with yourself in the process.

Chapter 7

Juiced Up

As I have mentioned throughout this book, making peace with food got me into a vibrational space where I could find the healthy eating style that works best for me. This all started to come together for me when I shifted my focus from weight loss to health.

Although I was feeling a wonderful sense of freedom after I quit dieting, and I was enjoying eating, physically I wasn't feeling great. From years of dieting, and all the stress surrounding it, my stomach hurt no matter what I ate unless I took an acid blocker—I had been on Prilosec for a number of years and finally decided I didn't want to take it anymore. Every time I tried to get off of it I was unsuccessful—the pain would come back. Basically, I was just covering up the problem but I didn't know what else to do.

I felt tired. I would get out to walk but I didn't have much energy for it. I wanted to try running but I couldn't imagine starting the way I was feeling. Sure, having all the extra weight wasn't helping, but I felt like it was something more than that.

One day I had a radical thought. *Is it possible I am not getting the proper nutrients?*

I know this may sound stupid but I had never thought about it before. My relationship with food had never been about nourishment. It had only been about calories, fat grams, points, or whatever it was I happened to be counting. My relationship with food was solely about weight.

I never thought much about my digestion either, and the fact that I couldn't seem to get off the acid blocker. It never occurred to me that perhaps I wasn't assimilating food properly. I was eating good quality, mostly organic food—*why did I still feel like shit?*

When I finally had this revelation, I talked to my friend David who had decided a few months before to replace going out to eat for lunch with a good quality, nutrient-dense powder he whipped up into a shake. He was feeling great and had even lost some weight—I decided to give it a go!

I used it for a month and didn't notice any change—I was still lacking energy and feeling poorly. In the meantime, I had stopped by this new juice bar that had opened in my town a few times, and tried some smoothies. Each time as I waited for it to be prepared I noticed, and read about, a three-day juice cleanse that they offered. It intrigued me ... and it scared me, so aside from noting it I did nothing more about it.

Right at this same time I started working with my new business coach. I was attempting to start a business using all the various certifications I had gotten, but I was really at a loss as to what it was going to look like, and on top of that I felt some sort of a disconnect about doing the work that I couldn't put my finger on.

Before we talked he had me fill out a lengthy questionnaire that covered all areas of life. When asked if I was happy with my current state of health and fitness, I talked about my dieting history and making peace with food. I mentioned that I would like to get to my natural size but that was about it. I didn't harp on it, or make it the focus of what I wanted to be working on.

For our first call together he called me from a conference that he was putting on with his brother. The guest speaker happened to be Frank Ferrante, who made the documentary film *May I Be Frank,* all about his total transformation from disease and overweight to health by going through a gratitude program *and* by eating a mostly raw diet with fresh pressed vegetable juices. After our call he sent me the documentary. It seemed kind of odd that he would send me this film when we had not discussed weight or health at all during our coaching call. Little did I know this seemingly random thing would change my life. I watched the documentary and Frank's transformation was so amazing.

I found myself at the juice place the very next day ordering the three-day cleanse!

This was on a Sunday and I was going to start the next day. I was having dinner at my friend Deb's house that night for some special occasion. She made beautiful filets and I had a few glasses of wine (OK, highly NOT recommended before going on a cleanse). Honestly, I knew absolutely nothing about juicing or doing any sort of a cleanse. I certainly didn't know that you were supposed to kind of lead up to it, lighten up your diet, and cut out caffeine and alcohol ... oops!

Actually, I think it was good that I didn't know anything about it. I had no expectations that it either might be terrible or amazing. The only thing that concerned me was the possibility of feeling starving. And, thankfully, that was not the case.

I say that it was good that I knew nothing about it because when you have expectations going into something, most times you will make those expectations come true. I found when I started coaching people to get started with juicing, if they had initial resistance before they even got started, even if they gave it a good go and had some pleasing results, it wouldn't stick. They would eventually fall into some version of the, "It's too hard," story and stop.

Being able to purchase the cleanse instead of making all the juice myself was fantastic for the first go round. I didn't get bogged down trying to figure out juice recipes and buying a shitload of produce. I did do that later on, but it was nice to get the taste of a juice cleanse in an easy fashion.

The cleanse I did consisted of four 16 oz. organic, fresh cold pressed vegetable and fruit juices, a small salad, a cup of vegan soup, kale chips, and an "emergency" cookie. The cookie was raw, vegan, no flour or sugar, and it tasted great, so I didn't wait for any emergency to eat it. I was ingesting something about every two hours, so not only was I not starving, I hardly got hungry.

And then, miracle of all miracles, I started to feel better, even after the first day. Juicing produce, as I came to learn more about, removes all of the insoluble fiber so there is little to no digestion involved. The juice was bypassing my troubled belly and the nutrients were getting absorbed easily. My body was getting nourished.

This was a profound thing for me. I had spent my whole teen and adult life battling with my body. Hating it. Not giving it what it needed. Starving it. Stuffing it. Wanting it to just go away.

Honestly, I never nourished myself on any level. Anything I did, whether it be exercise or, of course, what I ate or didn't eat, all boiled down to what would facilitate weight loss. I never thought about how I wanted to feel when I ate, or what exercise I might enjoy. I would just do whatever crazy diet and exercise plan I thought would get the weight off, until I couldn't do it anymore. Then I would regain the weight, to the point of hysteria, and start all over again.

******

This was an amazing time for me. For the first time in my life I was doing something to take care of myself, to nourish myself. I really wasn't thinking, *God, I hope this three-day cleanse helps me drop some weight.* I was just thrilled that I had started to feel better. I was thrilled that I was doing something good for myself; doing something good for my body and well-being. It wasn't punishing. It wasn't harsh. It was actually *beautiful.*

I had no problem doing the three days. In fact, I didn't want it to end. I was going to a friend's house on Martha's Vineyard on the fourth day so it wasn't really feasible to keep it going for the weekend. But I kept my eating pretty clean for the visit and the day after I got back I went out and bought a juicer.

I talked with one of the owners of the juice bar about whether I should get a juicer or a blender. We decided that, since I had enjoyed and had good results from the juice cleanse, I should just stick to juicing. I then inquired about where to find good juice recipes. She told me, "Just keep it simple. Start with celery, cucumber, and a couple of greens."

And so I did, and a few different variations of this juice have been my breakfast for the last several years. I call it the Screamin' Green juice—usually it is kale, collards (or another leafy green like chard or spinach), cucumber, celery, broccoli sprouts, and sometimes lemon. It's very green and takes a little getting used to, but I am so grateful for Screamin' Green because it was my catalyst to good health, and getting back to my natural weight.

I started juicing for breakfast and lunch and eating (for the most part) whole, nutrient-dense dinners. I began experimenting with food—eating different combinations of things to see what felt good in my stomach, and what gave me the most energy.

The important thing to note here is I DIDN'T TREAT IT LIKE A DIET. I was eating things that I knew had a lot of nutrients, and then experimenting with what felt the best for me. AND I didn't make it a rigid thing. If I was at a cookout I would eat the cookout food. If I went to dinner at a friend's I would eat what they were serving. Out to dinner I would often eat outside of my healthy eating plan because something looked delicious, and I was enjoying a relaxed evening with friends.

It was a new way of being for me. I was concerned with nourishment and feeling good. When I drank my Screamin' Green every morning I knew that I got a boatload of veggies and awesome nutrients in, so even if I had nothing green the rest of the day I was covered.

Some nice side effects came from all the juicing and whole food eating. My stomach issue resolved itself and pretty quickly and I was able to stop taking the Prilosec. My skin, which had been super red for years, cleared up. And I started to lose weight.

******

After I began getting into juicing, my coach sent me another documentary film—*Fat, Sick, and Nearly Dead*. This film was made by Joe Cross, an Australian man who also was very overweight, had a rare autoimmune disorder, and was on a lot of medications. He decided he was going to juice fast for 60 days and film the whole thing.

Again, he had incredible results, losing a lot of weight and reversing his health conditions. (Note: In both of these films they were supervised and monitored by a doctor—they did not go off any medications by themselves.)

This film got me thinking about what it would be like to do an all juice fast—maybe even for a week. I had been doing so much juicing that the idea didn't seem too daunting.

Then, one day, I was reading a post from Joel Runyon (The Blog of Impossible Things, Impossible HQ) about how he was going to team up with an organization called Pencils of Promise to raise $25,000 to build a school in Guatemala— they were calling it their Impossible Ones campaign. He challenged his community of readers to pick an impossible challenge themselves, and do a fundraiser around it.

I was often inspired by Joel's posts, but never did much about it. This post really stuck in my head, because the first thing that popped into my mind was *I could do a thirty-day juice fast.* But the more I thought about it, although it was definitely intimidating, I was pretty sure that I could do it. It wasn't like I had never juiced—I had been doing quite a bit of it, though I had never done a juice fast with no solid food.

Joel's challenge was, "Create your own impossible challenge – not just something you think you might be able to do. Pick something that scares you, that pushes your limits – that you might fail at. Then go do it, tell people about it and contribute to the Impossible School fund." I decided to add to my challenge—while doing the juice fast I would train for and run a 5-mile race (I was still pretty heavy and hadn't run in about 20 years). OK, that seemed to be impossible enough for me.

This was also awesome timing (well-orchestrated, Universe!) because it was mid-August, and I didn't have any social engagements in September; really I had nothing going on that month. And I found a 5-mile race just a few towns over the second to last day of the month. Perfect!

I woke up September first (after going out for a steak dinner the night before—what is wrong with me?) and started making juice. I drank four 16oz juices a day, sometimes five. I had my staples and then once a day I would experiment— that didn't always work out so well, especially when I decided to get into juicing a jalapeño. But generally they were all pretty good.

And I got out there and started pounding the pavement (literally—there was a lot of force landing on each one of those steps!). It was interesting because that was the part of the fundraiser that I didn't have confidence in. I *expected* it was going to be hard and, subsequently, it was. I only had a month—*This is going to be a disaster!*

I kept plodding along, but it was very slow getting any momentum going. I was getting frustrated with myself. It wasn't until I decided that I was just going to do the best that I could—and if I couldn't run the entire five miles by the end of the month I would just walk some of it and it would be no big deal—that I started to relax and gain some traction.

I was able to run about 2 ½ miles at a shot when it came time for the race. I hoped somehow adrenalin would kick in and I would be able to knock out the 5. I made it a little over 3 miles, about a 5K, before I had to stop and walk for a bit. Then I kind of walk/ran it (mostly walk) the rest of the way.

It was kind of slow going, but I finished pretty well—I was 91st ... out of 95. Luckily, I wasn't dead last so I didn't have the police car behind me with blue lights flashing, signaling the end of the race. I wanted to include the race photo with my last blog post about the month, but unfortunately it was hideous, so I had to have my friend Karen attest to the fact that I finished. She ran the race, won, had something to eat, got a pedicure, and then ran a ½ mile back to run me into the finish line. Somewhere in that last half mile was where the photo was snapped—it wasn't pretty. But I finished, and the challenge definitely got me on track to get in shape.

Juicing for a month, well, it was interesting. My stomach pain was completely gone, my skin looked great, and I lost more weight. I got used to the feeling of an empty stomach, so the only time I got into trouble was if I waited too long between juices—I would get irritable and start feeling really hungry. But the next juice would take care of it. I also drank coconut water with spirulina after running to get a little extra protein.

That's not the interesting part though. What was interesting was living for a month with food being taken out of the equation. No thinking about what I would have for dinner. No dinner preparation and sitting down to a meal. I did prepare most of my juices so that, of course, took up time. But the ritual of a meal was gone.

And beyond that, what was gone was a lot of my social life. I enjoy sharing meals or a glass of wine with friends—it is largely the way I stay connected. So instead I met friends for tea and walks. I was going to a meditation center, but that's pretty much just sitting in silence, so it wasn't much of a help socially. Truly it was the perfect opportunity to go inward, but I didn't take full advantage.

Honestly, I felt great, I felt crappy, I felt energized, I felt wicked tired, I felt excited, and sometimes I felt really sad.

When your body is not doing all the work of digestion, the digestive enzymes are freed up to clear out toxins stored in the body. And I can assure you, I had plenty of toxins stored up. So, as your body is detoxing it will cause some tiredness, and aches and pains. What I wasn't expecting was that this detoxing would also cause emotions to come to the surface. Hence the really sad feeling.

I couldn't even put my finger on what I was sad about. Finally, I went to the juice place to ask if this was normal—they told me it was.

But I have to admit, along with the sadness, I was also feeling a little disappointed. I had been reading about other people's experience with doing a juice fast, and some reported having this great feeling of intense clarity. Frankly, I was kind of looking forward to that. Instead, I was having some heavy periods of sadness—not what I was *expecting*.

In hindsight I see, as I said earlier, it would have been a good time to go inward. It would have been a good time to meditate daily, rather than just going to the center once a week. It would have been a good time to do yoga and to spend time at the beach and in the woods.

I say this, though, as a reflection, and not a "should have". My experience was absolutely perfect just the way it was. It was life changing. I started running, which was something I had wanted to do for years. I regained good health, which is priceless. And I really started writing my blog as I chronicled the month. I had been so timid about posting. This gave me the opportunity—since I was fundraising I wanted to document my progress for those who donated. That, again, is priceless to me, as is the fact that this journey has culminated in this book. I am so grateful to have had the whole experience.

******

Aside from the challenge, another reason I wanted to do an extended juice fast was to determine whether or not I would recommend it to others. My results were pretty profound so, in that sense, yes, I would recommend it, especially for someone who has a lot of weight they would like to transmute, or health issues they are really struggling with (of course under a doctor's supervision).

But would I say it was necessary? No. I got great results before and after the fast with my health and weight loss. What I would highly recommend to anyone interested in better health, and perhaps getting back to their naturally thin size, is to do some sort of three or five-day cleanse.

Don't panic! This doesn't necessarily have to involve juicing if it's not your bag. Juicing worked great for me and still does, but I finally had to come to the realization that it is not for everybody, despite my initial wish to push it on everyone I came across. You can do a smoothie cleanse, a raw food cleanse, or simply eliminate all processed foods. There are many routes to take; there is no one "right" way.

For anyone interested in making a change, I would love for you to do this because it will get you back in touch with your body. When you do a cleanse it infuses your body with nutrition, and it gets rid of any cravings you might have for sugary and processed food. Plus, it starts to eliminate stored toxins that cause problems in our systems. Afterward, you are truly able to listen to your body, and hear what it really wants and needs to eat.

The only things I craved when I was doing the fast, and waited too long between juices, were sushi and roasted broccoli. I never thought I would hear myself say, "I'm dying for some broccoli!" But now I crave it all the time—it's one of my favorite foods to eat.

Also, if you have any kind of digestion problems, doing a cleanse is going to help. Your body needs to be able to assimilate food properly in order for you to regain health and get back to your natural size.

But the best thing about all of this cleansing business is that it will lead you to finding the healthy eating style that works best for you. Imagine how you would feel if your body was truly nourished. If you are anything like I was, you may never have had this experience before. I found that, when I started caring for my body with nourishing foods, I started to take care of myself in other ways as well. It turned the tide from me being constantly at war with myself to finding an inner peace that radiated out into my whole life.

Believe me, even if you have some trepidation with the idea of a "cleanse", just refer to it as something else, like a warm shower for your insides, because it is totally worth it.

Chapter 8

Whole, Nutrient-Dense Eating

Many years ago, I lived in a tiny, one-bedroom apartment. The kitchen was, I guess, what you would call a galley kitchen, but it was more like the galley of the smallest boat on Earth. Because it was so small it had mini appliances—the freezer was just a tiny box inside the fridge that would ice over. I was constantly chipping away at that thing with a knife and a hammer because I had to make more room for my life blood—frozen diet dinners.

I actually felt pretty good about myself when I was at the grocery store and those frozen delights were the only thing in my cart. I figured I must look pretty healthy ... because I equated health solely with weight loss.

Another example of my distorted view of healthy eating was my surprise 20-something birthday party. The gag gifts were all fat free "food" items, because my friends knew that was all I ate (and a shitload of napkins because I had this quirky thing about not being able to eat without a napkin). That was kind of a weird birthday looking back on it, but it was indicative of how strongly I believed that anything without fat (although laden with sugar and everything artificial) was good for me to eat. When my friends tried to think of ridiculous things to get me, that's what they thought of. What is funny about it to me now is my skewed perception and the way I clung to it so tightly.

You wouldn't catch me eating a salad because the only salad dressings I liked had a lot of fat in them. I'm not really a stupid person, although it's sure sounding that way right now. I could have researched nutrition, micronutrients and such but the truth is I didn't care about it. I didn't care about my actual health at all. My only concern about what I was putting into my body was the fat gram count.

When I joined Weight Watchers, my final diet, I affectionately referred to it as the caffeine and nicotine diet. Basically, I drank a ton of coffee and smoked a million cigarettes to stave off hunger between my little faux food meals.

It was around this time that I started to have panic attacks again. It was devastating because it was something I thought I had conquered years ago. It didn't occur to me that maybe the panic might have had something to do with all the caffeine and nicotine that was coursing through my body.

It took me some time after I quit dieting to actually think about how what I ingested affected the way I felt. It took me getting to the point where I really felt pretty lousy to start doing some investigation.

******

When I say investigation, I am not talking about researching the latest nutritional trends. I am an avid reader and enjoy reading up on these topics but I found that there were vast discrepancies between what different experts would recommend as the way we should be eating for optimal health.

Some claim that animal products are the root of all evil. Others ban all grains in favor of animal protein—it's the way our ancient ancestors ate so we should be eating that way too. Then there are the studies of different cultures and their health rates—some experts claim that everyone on Earth should be eating the way one culture does. Reading all these different accounts didn't make any sense.

This led me to the brilliant conclusion (OK, we all can easily conclude this) that I have been proclaiming throughout this book—there is no one right way to eat. There just isn't. It's not possible, as what feels right to me one day might even change the next. Not only is there no one right way for everyone, the right way for each of us morphs over time. And when I say *right* I mean the foods that feel best in our bodies and that we enjoy eating.

******

One thing that I did find to be consistent among the experts in nutrition was this—**eat whole, nutrient-dense foods.** Meaning food that is as close to its natural state as possible.

Such a simple thing and something that finally made sense to me. Eat things that are whole; that haven't been processed much. Yes, everything we buy in the store is processed to some degree because it has to be harvested, packaged, and shipped. Most of us are not in the situation where we can just walk out to our back yard and harvest the day's meals. But we can be choosey about what we buy in the store, and, if available, shop at local farms.

You know what is not on the list of whole, nutrient-dense food? Frozen diet dinners. Nor are most things that come in a box, and things that have more than one ingredient. Try reading the ingredients on some of these boxed and diet foods—it will make your head spin.

When I finished my first three-day juice cleanse I was so excited about the way I felt. Not only was I already feeling physically better, I also didn't have any cravings for sugary food. I wanted to eat more vegetables—my body was now sending me signals that told me what it really wanted and needed to eat, instead of me continually setting it up to crave more sugary and processed food that didn't provide any nutrition.

So, it made sense to me that the foundation of my healthy eating plan would be vegetables and some fruit. Then I started to experiment—what did I want to be eating with my veggies?

I simply ate different things and checked out how I felt. Historically, I knew that beans don't usually sit well in my stomach, although I love the taste and consistency of them. So, logically, beans were not going to be a staple in my own plan, even though there are people who thrive on eating a lot of beans.

I tried out having whole grains as a staple but found they sometimes didn't work that well in my system. Dairy seemed to be OK but I felt better eating it in smaller amounts than I used to, and goat dairy worked out even better. Fish, poultry, and red meat all sit well with me as do nuts and seeds. I never was that crazy about eating tofu and other soy products so they were out as well. I was really excited about juicing so green juice was definitely staying in the mix.

After taking some time to experiment I had it—in the moment I had what I call my 90% healthy eating style. I say 90% because we don't solely live inside the vacuum of our own homes. There are parties, and holidays, and times when we just feel like having a piece of cake. Again, as I want to really stress this point, **there is nothing wrong with eating outside of the guidelines you have come up with.**

They are just that—guidelines. Guidelines for a way of eating that make you feel optimal. You are not putting yourself on yet another diet. You are finding a way to eat that you love, and that you will continue with because it is awesome and it feels great. It is not something to endure because it sucks.

Also, I say 90%—is it always a solid 90% for me? No. Sometimes it's more like 80%. It dips below that at times as well. When I'm on vacation and not preparing any of my own food it certainly does. And sometimes I just feel like eating a bowl of pasta, so I do. It's not about deprivation.

Throughout this process of first quitting dieting and then coming up with my 90ish% healthy eating style, I also gave thought to where I wanted to source the food I was eating. I was juicing a lot of my vegetables so I felt strongly about having the vegetables I juice be organic, as I think the pesticides become more concentrated when vegetables are juiced. As for eating veggies, I try for mostly organic, but I'm OK with going outside of that when it's not available or it's wildly more expensive.

I feel physically better eating animal protein, but I am also an animal lover, so it is important to me to buy humanely raised. I am fortunate to have local farms nearby that sell their own meat, and I can get fresh organic eggs from my CSA, where I can see the chickens hanging out enjoying themselves in the yard. By the way, if you have any CSA (Community Supported Agriculture) programs available near you, it is a great way to get super fresh, local produce at a great price.

But, in saying all of this, sometimes I don't have control over where the food I am eating is sourced. So if I choose to eat out, go to a party, or anything like that, I have to be OK with it—again a matter of *feel good about what you eat*. I don't get stressed out—I just have gratitude for the veggies, and whatever else that is served, that gave their life to sustain me. Thank you.

These are just my preferences—we all have different budgets, different food availability, and different beliefs. Remember, you must feel good about what you eat. So I invite you to, in addition to investigating what foods feel best in your body, give thought to what feels best for you regarding where your food comes from.

******

Are you ready to find your own healthy eating style? Take a pause right now and really think about this, because you may not be. This book chronicles the process I went through to regain health and my natural size. And it was a process. If you are reading this and still happen to be in the throes of dieting, doing a cleanse and investigating your own healthy eating style might be reminiscent to you of just going on another diet, and it is very important for me to convey that this is not what this book is about. It is not about finding a quick fix so you can knock off those extra pounds before your friend's wedding. It's about finding peace with something that you may have been battling with for most of your life, and then coming from that peaceful place to find the way of eating that nourishes and sustains you in the best possible way.

So if you find yourself reading the last section of this book feeling like you want to cry because it seems like I am suggesting you do something restrictive that is not my intent. After teaching a class, I had a woman come up to me and say, "What you are doing is just another diet." It was said with an angry tone, somewhat on the verge of tears. So I feel the need to say at this juncture that you may not be ready to take this step yet.

At this point you might just need to practice eating in a peaceful way whatever it is you are eating because, truly, making peace with food is the critical factor. If you haven't taken that step, nothing I am talking about in this last section will fall into place.

It is a process, and when you first find peace with food, and peace with yourself wherever you are in the moment, your healthy eating style will pretty much find you. Mine did, but it didn't happen the minute after I stopped dieting.

This is a time to be really gentle with yourself. It is a time to nourish yourself, maybe for the first time in your life. It is a time to feel alive in the amazing body you are in right now. It is a time to flourish.

******

So whenever you are feeling ready to do some sleuthing to find a way of eating that best supports you, here are some suggestions on where to start. Going back to the notion of whole, nutrient-dense eating, it seems that the foundation of a healthy eating style would be vegetables, whole fruits, good quality fats, nuts, and seeds (unless of course you have an intolerance or allergy).

Remember, this is NOT ANOTHER DIET. It is a new way of being with food, focusing on finding foods that will nourish you physically and emotionally. If you have practiced one form or another of calorie restriction for most of your life, and have lived by the calories in calories out mantra, consider this—are all calories the same? Are 200 calories of broccoli going to do the same thing in your body as 200 calories of soda? I think, without citing any science backup, we can all logically agree that the broccoli will provide needed nutrients and fiber whereas the soda will just dump a bunch of sugar in our system. 200 calories of broccoli = a LOT of broccoli—you might not be able to eat that much in one sitting. Finding your healthy eating style requires changing your focus from light, low cal, low fat "foods" to nutrient packed, real, whole foods. Again, logically doesn't the latter seem like a better idea?

Also, just a note on fat. I know I held a belief that fat makes you fat for most of my life. We have been conditioned to believe that eating fat puts fat on our bodies. I am by no means a nutritionist, but good quality fats (like olive oil, coconut oil, avocado, and nuts) are essential nutrients for us. If you happen to be holding on to a fear of eating anything that has a fat gram count, you may want to do a little research so you can lay that belief to rest. I wanted to mention this here because I have seen this fear cause hesitation for many people when I suggest whole, nutrient dense eating.

OK, now it is time for you to have some fun—and, yes, this should be fun! First, are there any foods you know you have a hard time digesting? For now, leave those foods out. Things may change and you might add them back in later, but for now, if it doesn't make you feel good leave it out—like me and the beans.

Then just start eating! Consciously eat different whole foods and notice how they make you feel—make sure to notice how they feel on all levels. For instance, someone may be able to digest meat just fine, but emotionally doesn't feel good about eating it. The foods you are eating should feel good in all ways.

See how whole grains make you feel (eating the grain in its most natural form instead of transformed into bread or pasta). How about whole milk dairy? Cow's milk versus goat or sheep milk? If you choose to eat them, how do fish, poultry, or red meat make you feel? Eggs? Tofu or tempeh?

You can also experiment with food combining. Sometimes a food on its own won't cause an issue for you but combined with something else it will. For me, I am better off eating fruit by itself or with a few nuts—it digests better that way.

If you did a juice or smoothie cleanse how was that for you? If drinking juice or smoothies made you feel good, try keeping it up. Is it fun for you to come up with exotic combinations? Great! Or maybe you just have one in particular you want to have every day—like me and my Screamin' Green. Do you enjoy the process of juicing or blending?

Now is also a great time to experiment with cooking. You can try out new recipes or concoct some of your own. Do you enjoy cooking something elaborate or keeping it simple?

Does combining a lot of different flavors taste good to you, or do you prefer the taste to be simple? Do you like cooking a big batch of something and eating it for several days, or do you like to have more of a variety?

I found that I like keeping it pretty simple, and I tend to eat the same things over and over again. I like to do a salad, a cooked vegetable, and some sort of protein. One of my favorites is kale salad, roasted broccoli, and a piece of salmon. But then, once in a while, I'll take a bunch of time and make something more elaborate like ground turkey and eggplant stew with a roasted red pepper tahini sauce over cauliflower "rice".

I'm hoping you can see that this really is a fun process, and that you will enjoy your investigation. Yes, there will be some flops along the way as you find things that don't agree with you, or you will try to wing a dish combining things that you think will go together, and then you'll dig in only to find they don't go together at all. It's OK—it's all part of the process of finding foods that you enjoy preparing and eating, and that feel optimal in your system.

******

Imagine eating food that makes you feel good physically and emotionally in a conscious, peaceful way. For me it was such a radical shift from my frenzied eating while dieting; eating things I didn't enjoy much and hardly being aware I was eating, always wanting something more. Now when I eat I am satisfied. I feel nourished. I feel whole—whether what I ate falls into my 90% healthy eating style or not.

Chapter 9

Peaceful Is the New Normal?

As I sit down to write this final chapter, we are coming to the end of yet another year.

It seems to always catch me by surprise. Thus, this thought starts to sneak up as well when the holidays approach—*What have I accomplished this year?*

Then, unsurprisingly, my thoughts usually go to the things I haven't accomplished yet, or the projects that didn't turn out as planned. My mind goes to the things that I *should* have done.

Cue *Auld Lang Syne*, and all of us running for our notebooks to write a list of resolutions for the New Year.

I think I say this in one way or another every year—**New Year's resolutions are bullshit!** They are, for most people, likely a list of the things they think they should be doing. It's like ending the year with a big slap in the face— *Why haven't you been doing these things already?*

It's akin to starting a diet—we begin enthusiastically, and then a week or two into it we realize this is NOT what we want to be doing. It's something we think we should be doing, but it definitely sucks and we really want to stop doing it. A battle ensues in our mind—Should vs. Want, with Guilt as the moderator. Eventually, Want punches Should out, and then runs amuck fueled by Guilt's taunting.

Following suit, we start the year doing our list of shoulds (probably going on a diet is one of them) and stick with it for a couple of weeks. Usually within that time we realize, as with the diet, that these things are NOT what we want to be doing. Most likely we quit doing them, and we get to start the New Year feeling like a big loser. What an awesome way to commence!

Instead, what if on New Year's Day we made a list of our dreams? What if we made a list of the things we would love to do in the coming year? And what if we accepted exactly how our lives are in this moment as we start the New Year? What if we skipped berating ourselves for the things we didn't accomplish, and just started working on our dreams from exactly where we are, without any judgment?

Now *that* would be an awesome way to commence the New Year!

I don't know about you, but I am done waging war against myself. Although it was a long one, I love that my journey with food, weight, and dieting ultimately taught me how to live a peaceful life. I absolutely had to accept where I was, quite overweight, and then I had to stop labeling myself and whatever food I was ingesting as "good" or "bad"; I had to stop the judgment.

After spending most of my life battling with my body, and with what I was or was not eating, when I removed that stressor it was like I was living in a whole new world. Then, kind of by osmosis, I started to approach my entire life this way. I accepted where I was in all areas of my life to be exactly where I am supposed to be in this moment, and I stopped putting focus on the things I thought to be lacking, and, of course, blaming myself for that lack.

It's as if someone was literally punching me in the face every day and then they stopped. It was such a relief! And although I still have some blips from time to time, this peaceful place has now become my new normal.

Is now the time for you to find a new normal?

******

To be happy. Isn't this why we do a lot of what we do, because we want to be happy? I know that for a good part of my life I thought my happiness rested on being a particular weight. Certainly I would be happy when I was thin.

During my decades of dieting I definitely experienced times when I was thin. Sometimes even super thin. Guess what? I still didn't feel happy. There was always something that could be better; I could be more muscular, I could be even thinner, I could have a better shaped ass.

Being thin did not produce a feeling of happiness within me. Sure, I had some fleeting moments of feeling victorious—I had defeated the enemy ... at least temporarily. But I didn't feel happy because I still didn't accept myself the way I was. And I worried—when was the other shoe going to drop? When was I going to start gaining the weight back?

When you are constantly worried, you aren't going to feel happy, no matter how thin you get. After I stopped dieting, eventually I stopped worrying about my weight. It was what it was—I accepted it.

This made me realize something—I was used to being worried.

I grew up worrying. Since it was something that started at a young age the pattern easily wired into my brain. It was more "normal" for me to feel worried and anxious than it was to feel happy.

I have actually caught myself, at times when I was feeling happy about something, suddenly feeling jarred by this and frantically searching my brain for what I should be worrying about. I would feel guilty about feeling happy, like I was cheating on my anxiety in some way.

I didn't realize that I was not very familiar with this happy feeling. It felt good, but it didn't feel normal. This would prompt my mind to look for what it was used to, regardless of whether that state of mind was pleasant or not. As with changing thoughts and beliefs about food and my body, I realized that I would also have to *train myself* to feel happy.

Not too long ago I had a situation happening in my life that I became very worried about. At the same time I had a lot of wonderful things happening, but I wouldn't let myself enjoy the good things because I was so focused on what wasn't working. I clung to it, desperate to make it somehow click, instead of just letting it go and seeing all the good things before me.

As I feared, the thing I was worried about finally came crumbling down around me. When it did, all the worry and stress I had been feeling for months manifested into me getting quite physically sick—we are powerful creators!

But despite that, once I finally calmed down and started to see other options, I was so grateful not to be experiencing that level of stress anymore. I was able to actually see and start experiencing the good things that were happening, which had been there all along. Sure, there were still many things I could have been worrying about, but instead I just felt content with what was.

Just like when I dieted for so many years—it clearly wasn't working as I continued to gain more and more weight. As painful and stressful as this pattern was, it was again something I started doing as a child. It felt familiar and normal.

Quitting dieting and just eating was so unfamiliar to me that every time I tried I couldn't do it. I would eventually find myself back on another diet and feeling all the painful, yet familiar feelings that go along with it. I finally had to train myself to stop dieting, and did it feel good once it became familiar!

Feelings are habitual.

The body gets used to the chemical reactions our feelings cause and it looks to recreate what it knows. Whether they serve us or not, the patterns get wired into our brains.

Being happy is just like anything else—all it takes is making a conscious choice and then building a new habit. I learned how to do this by training myself to be peaceful around food. Then I made the conscious choice to focus on what was working and good in my life, and I practiced that until it began to feel familiar.

So happiness, like everything else in life, is a practice. It's a choice. I can choose to put it off—to wait until some elusive time like, *When I'm thin enough*—or I can choose to be happy right now, at whatever size I happen to be.

To me this is a really exciting prospect. So very simple but it is the absolute truth. It's my choice. Even though my brain was wired with certain beliefs about food, diet, and my body, I still have the choice to change them.

This didn't happen overnight. There was the part of me that wanted to cling to these beliefs—it was what I knew, and believed to be true, despite the mounting evidence to the contrary. It was the way I had always perceived things, and, frankly, the way a hell of a lot of other people perceived food, diet, and body image. Who was I to step outside of this box?

But as I looked around, this way of thinking really didn't seem to be working out very well for any of the people in my camp. They all seemed to be miserable about it, whether they were what might be perceived as thin or overweight. I didn't really know many people who were happy with their relationship with food or their relationship with their body.

My choice wasn't a popular one. Although people seemed to be miserable in their beliefs, my choice to stop dieting flew in the face of them. It freaked people out. It almost seemed to make some people mad—*How can you be doing this? What about your health?*

As I've said, initially this was very difficult for me. I always longed to fit in and never really felt like I did. Now here I was, way overweight, and not on a diet. More than that, I wasn't joining any of the conversations about dieting, and being "good" or "bad". I wasn't lamenting about my weight to other people.

But as I persevered, training myself to have more positive and expansive beliefs, it felt so good that I didn't care about fitting in that way anymore. I didn't care what other people thought. I was in love in a new relationship—a new relationship with food.

******

I was finally able to find the joy of eating. Not fleeting moments of joy followed by regret and remorse, but sustained joy from the act of eating food.

Before I quit dieting, sometimes I would have some joy eating a favorite food. But that would quickly turn ugly after I was done. Most likely I overate the favorite food, so I would feel physically ill. Then my thoughts would turn to fear and guilt, and, of course, I would have some awful things to say to myself.

I was stepping away from an abusive relationship with food, and with myself.

I think now about how many things unrelated to food or diet I didn't step away from because they were familiar— jobs I hated, relationships that clearly weren't working, business partnerships that were falling apart. I would do anything in my power to force these things to work, feeling totally miserable, simply because they were known. Trying something different, something unknown, scared the bejesus out of me.

Stepping outside of my known beliefs about food taught me something very valuable. It taught me that the unknown can be awesome!

******

I didn't know how it was going to happen, but I found a place deep inside of me that trusted that the weight would come off organically, naturally. As I write this now, I see what I actually found was myself.

I found my true self—the part of me that remembers that everything is actually OK. The part of me that is not fearful, not panicked, not worn out by constant stress. I found my home, my light; I found a whole new way of inhabiting this body.

I found a life that is not ruled by fear.

I am sitting here now feeling grateful and kind of amazed— amazed at all the things I have done since I made that initial leap into the unknown and quit dieting:

I started a business with a friend.

When that fell apart I started my own business, even though I didn't really know what that business was going to be.

I took several trainings.

I hired an awesome coach.

I went to Toastmasters to learn how to public speak (OK, this was under duress of the aforementioned awesome coach, but **I did it** and completed my competent communicator award).

I started juicing.

I did a thirty-day juice fast.

I started running (while doing the juice fast).

I started my blog.

I actually published blog posts and a few people read them.

I started telling people about my blog posts and more people read them.

I found a way of eating that totally supports me.

I lost the weight easily and organically.

I coached other people.

I developed classes and taught them.

I traveled throughout the county by myself.

I attended conferences.

I spoke at a conference!

I wrote most of a book that didn't see the light of day.

I wrote and submitted two book proposals.

AND ... **I wrote a book and published it!** (Well, by the time you are reading this the statement will be true).

These were all things that were totally unknown to me, and most of them normally would have scared me to the point of not even considering them as options. But I was now in a place where I didn't have to know how things were going to happen. I had found the part of me that just trusted that, if I put myself out there, things would happen in exactly the right way.

There were many times when things that I tried completely fell apart. Only now I was able to recover—I didn't let myself fall apart in the process. I was able to see pretty quickly that it was for the best, and it always led me to the next best thing. Even though there are still times when I start to get a sliver of doubt, that place in me that trusts is strong enough to quiet it down; to not let it get out of hand.

That place of trust in me has allowed me to try things that are way outside my comfort zone. Things that I thought I would never do. Things that just seemed way too scary. That place in me has allowed me to write this book, which has always been an unrealized dream, not knowing exactly how I am going to get anyone to read it. That place in me gave me faith that I just have to show up, to keep moving in a direction, and the Universe will take care of the rest.

I am so grateful now for the pain of my years of dieting and weight gain because, when the pain became too much, it finally got me to open a new door, a door to a place I didn't know, but the unknown became OK. It allowed me to forge a new path, first with food, and subsequently in all areas of my life. It got me to realize that doing something that is known and miserable sucks a lot more that doing something that is initially unknown. There is still some fear from time to time, but not the pervasive fear that used to be my life.

As you know, this journey I went on, changing my thoughts and beliefs about food, diet, and body image and finding the eating style that best supports me, leading me to get back to my natural size and good health, took some time. It didn't happen in the blink of an eye.

I had to take the time to train myself to find new normals. I had to decide what I wanted that normal to be, and I had to choose to go in that direction. I am writing this book with the hope and faith that it will serve as a springboard for you to leap into your own unknowns; to find your new normals.

This process is absolutely worth whatever time it takes. There is no better gift I could have ever given myself than that day I finally banished dieting for good. So many things spilled forth from it, and my life continues to get better and better.

I can truly say, "I love my life!" and it is not just a platitude. Finding peace with food led me down the path to a peaceful, joyful life.

Please discover for yourself the joy of eating. Who knows where it might take you.

Afterword

I feel like this book has always been inside of me—even when I was at my heaviest. The problem was when I was at my heaviest, even though I knew somehow I was going to lose the weight and then hopefully help others by sharing what I learned, I couldn't help others until I helped myself.

We hear a lot about self-care these days, but I know for me it always sounded like just a nice idea. I never put much time or effort into caring for myself because my belief system of *not good enough* always overrode any effort I would make.

When I actually started to take care of myself, simply by wondering one day if I was getting the proper nutrients for optimal health, it was like a floodlight illuminated allowing me to finally see clearly. All of my life I have aspired to be of service to others, not realizing my effectiveness was greatly diminished by not taking care of myself first.

It came as a surprise to me as I wrote this book how much being kind to myself around food and my body, and wanting to take care of myself, changed my entire life. As I was reading through it again I saw that I mentioned this a lot, the peace I have found through this process, and I wondered if it was too repetitive. But I realized I kept saying it because I kept finding anew as I was writing what a profound effect this journey to weight loss and health has had on me. It has been about **so** much more than weight loss.

Yes, it was exciting to lose the weight in a way that was a joy, not a hardship. But when I started to focus my coaching practice on weight loss, my own weight loss turned into a "should". I started worrying about my weight again and it became physically apparent.

I took a break from the weight loss gig to work on another project and my clothes started fitting normally again—what I was working on didn't feel contingent upon what size my body was.

When the project I was working on went in a different direction than I planned, I wrote this book.

You know what sucks about writing a book on how you lost the weight and kept it off? You start worrying about keeping it off so you can promote the damn book.

You know what happens when you start worrying about gaining weight? You put your jeans on after wearing yoga pants all winter and say, "Shit, this is not how I remember these pants fitting ... and it's not because they are too loose."

This is so interesting to me when I can look at it as an observer rather than as my old weight-obsessed self.

The latter whispers words like *you're a fraud* in my ear.

But simply as an observer I can see exactly what is happening—it illustrates the whole premise of this book, and how I lost weight in the first place. When you feel at peace with food and with your body, at whatever size it happens to be in the moment, you are in vibrational alignment to enjoy the healthy eating style that is optimal for you, and any excess weight will take care of itself.

When you are feeling stressed and judgmental about food and your body it's a different story. Feeling stressed actually prompts your body to hold on to weight, and at the same time it does nothing to help you employ some self-care strategies that you know intellectually would get you right back to feeling energized and light.

When I let my observer-self shine through, it simply asked, "Why?"

Why am I not taking care of myself right now?

The answer: because I am about to put something I have created out into the world, and despite the fact that I felt pretty good about what I was producing as I was writing it, now that it is going to become a reality, old, shitty, *not good enough* thoughts are sneaking in while I'm not looking. And they are having a ball wreaking havoc with my system.

This could be a great time for me to self-destruct and throw away everything I've worked on, and a huge dream in the process. My old self would likely take the opportunity and bail, running an unending loop of thoughts like, *You have no idea what you are doing. Who is going to listen to you anyway? No one is going to read this—it sucks. No, you suck.*

But, thankfully, that peaceful place I found within myself as I have gone through this journey to weight loss and health still holds strong. It can reside with the doubts and fears that pop in unannounced, and it keeps me moving forward despite them.

So my fondness for wearing "activewear", and in turn being anything but active, need not be a sign of my impending demise. It's just a nudge, reminding me that I am actually OK, that everything is actually OK, when I let go of the angst and come back to that peaceful place. It's a nudge to take care of myself because I deserve it, not to prove anything to myself or anyone else, but simply for that reason alone.

And you deserve it too!

Writing this book was so wonderful because it reiterated for me the importance of being kind and nurturing to ourselves; the importance of really taking care of and loving ourselves; the importance of caring about feeling good. Switching my focus from weight loss to health—to feeling better by nourishing myself—that's when everything came together for me. That's when I got to the place where I can perhaps be of service to others, because I took care of myself first.

You deserve every good thing no matter what size or shape your body happens to be in this moment. You deserve to be cared for. You deserve to be treated with kindness and respect. Instead of waiting for some future time when you think you are more deserving, please know that you are deserving right NOW. And the only person you can rely on to treat you this way is you.